D1739288

HUMAN GROWTH HORMONE

HUMAN GROWTH HORMONE

Progress and Challenges

edited by

Louis E. Underwood
University of North Carolina
School of Medicine
Chapel Hill, North Carolina

Marcel Dekker, Inc.   **New York and Basel**

Library of Congress Cataloging-in-Publication Data

Human growth hormone.

Based on presentations made at a symposium sponsored
by Genentech, Inc. in Apr. 1986.
   Includes bibliographies and index.
   1. Somatotropin--Physiological effect--Congresses.
2. Somatotropin--Therapeutic use--Congresses.
I. Underwood, Louis E.
III. Genentech, Inc. [DNLM: 1. Somatotropin--congresses.
WK 515 H9181 1986]
QP572.S6H86   1988   612'.6   87-24463
ISBN 0-8247-7813-8

MARCEL DEKKER, INC.
270 Madison Avenue, New York, New York 10016

Current printing (last digit):
10 9 8 7 6 5 4 3 2 1

PRINTED IN THE UNITED STATES OF AMERICA

To

Alvin B. Hayles, M.D., Emeritus Professor of Pediatrics, Mayo Medical School, Rochester, Minnesota, pioneer in pediatric endocrinology and a beloved colleague and friend

James M. Tanner, M.D., Emeritus Professor of Growth and Development, Institute of Child Health, London, who has transformed the knowledge of the auxologist/ anthropologist into a form that is useful to physicians caring for children with growth disorders

Alfred E. Wilhelmi, D.Phil., Emeritus Professor of Biochemistry, Emory University, Atlanta, Georgia, whose tireless efforts have made it possible for thousands of growth hormone-deficient children to grow.

Preface

In the three decades since growth hormone (GH) was first isolated, steady progress has been made in defining this peptide's physicochemical properties, direct and indirect biological actions, receptor–ligand interactions, and genomic structure. As new laboratory techniques were developed, they have been applied readily to the study of GH, with the result that one of the first RIAs developed was for GH, the gene for GH and related peptides were among the first encoding for hormones to be characterized, and large-scale production of recombinant human GH was preceded only by the production of insulin. Despite these advances, progress in studies of GH as a therapeutic agent have been slowed by the lack of sufficient supplies of pure peptide. The consequence of this GH famine, therefore, is that clinical research has lagged behind laboratory investigation. For example, GH is recognized as a potent anabolic agent that stimulates indirectly the synthesis of DNA, RNA, and proteins, and promotes cell proliferation and nitrogen retention. Nevertheless, the applications of these insights to the treatment of human disease have been limited almost entirely to the treatment of children who have delayed statural growth due to GH deficiency. Little information is available about the effects of GH on conditions in which its anabolic effects might be beneficial. With the availability of recombinant GH in abundance, new opportunities will emerge to study this hormone, and particularly to determine whether GH has additional clinical uses.

The contributions in this volume are derived from presentations made at a symposium on GH sponsored by Genentech, Inc., and held in April 1986. Current understanding of the direct and indirect actions of GH are reviewed, as are recent insights into some of the mechanisms of GH action and the nature of interactions between GH and its receptor. The wide divergence of opinions about which children might (or might not) benefit from GH therapy is made obvious by the discussion in Chapter 7 of controversies in the treatment of short-stature children. Major problems are the ethics of treating children outside controlled trials when the likelihood for benefit and the potential for side effects are not known fully, and the possible adverse psychological effects when therapy is unsuccessful or is less successful than anticipated. Also still to be settled are the questions of whether the short-term benefits of GH will be sustained with long-term therapy and whether there will be late side effects of therapy. Some of the presentations at this symposium were also intended to focus on possible uses of GH for treatment of conditions other than short stature. Studies of this nature are in their infancy, but I hope that presentation of the rationale for trials and preliminary results in several conditions will stimulate the reader to follow the progress of future investigations.

Louis E. Underwood

Contents

Contributors

John F. Aloia, M.D. Chairman, Department of Medicine, Winthrop–University Hospital, Mineola, New York

Arthur J. Ammann, M.D. Director, Department of Collaborative Medical Research, Genentech, Inc., South San Francisco, California

Gary Balian, Ph.D. Professor, Departments of Orthopedics and Biochemistry, University of Virginia School of Medicine, Charlottesville, Virginia

Barry B. Bercu, M.D. Professor, Department of Pediatrics, University of South Florida College of Medicine, St. Petersburg, Florida

Robert M. Blizzard, M.D. Director, Children's Medical Center, Department of Pediatrics, University of Virginia School of Medicine, Charlottesville, Virginia

Samuel J. Casella, M.D.* Clinical Instructor, Division of Endocrinology, Department of Pediatrics, University of North Carolina School of Medicine, Chapel Hill, North Carolina

David R. Clemmons, M.D. Associate Professor, Department of

Current affiliation
*Assistant Professor, Division of Endocrinology, Department of Pediatrics, Johns Hopkins University School of Medicine, Baltimore, Maryland

Medicine, University of North Carolina School of Medicine, Chapel Hill, North Carolina

Jean Closset, Ph.D. First Assistant, Department of Medicine, University of Liege, Liege, Belgium

Stanton H. Cohn, Ph.D.* Senior Scientist, Medical Research Center, Brookhaven National Laboratories, Upton, New York

Pierre De Meyts, M.D. Director, Department of Diabetes, Endocrinology and Metabolism, City of Hope National Medical Center, Duarte, California

James Frane, Ph.D. Senior Statistical Analyst, Department of Clinical Research, Genentech, Inc., South San Francisco, California

S. Douglas Frasier, M.D. Professor, Department of Pediatrics, University of California at Los Angeles School of Medicine, Los Angeles, and Chief, Department of Pediatrics, Olive View Medical Center, Sylmar, California

H. Maurice Goodman, Ph.D. Professor and Chairman, Department of Physiology, and Associate Dean for Scientific Affairs, University of Massachusetts Medical School, Worcester, Massachusetts

Erela Gorin† Visiting Associate Professor, Department of Physiology, University of Massachusetts Medical School, Worcester, Massachusetts

Harvey J. Guyda, M.D., F.R.C.P.(C) Director, Division of Endocrinology and Metabolism, Department of Pediatrics, Montreal Children's Hospital, and Professor of Pediatrics and Medicine, McGill University, Montreal, Quebec, Canada

Georges P. Hennen, M.D., Ph.D. Professor of Endocrinology, Department of Medicine, University of Liege, Liege, Belgium

Raymond L. Hintz, M.D. Professor, Department of Pediatrics, Stanford University School of Medicine, Stanford, California

---

Current affiliation
*Consulting Professor, Department of Medicine, Stanford University School of Medicine, Stanford, California
†Senior Lecturer, Department of Biochemistry, Faculty of Medicine, Technion, Haifa, Israel

Thomas W. Honeyman, Ph.D. Associate Professor, Department of Physiology, University of Massachusetts Medical School, Worcester, Massachusetts

Mary Hynes, B.S. Curriculum in Neurobiology, Department of Physiology, University of North Carolina School of Medicine, Chapel Hill, North Carolina

M. Mapoko Ilondo University of Leuven School of Medicine, Leuven, Belgium

Ann J. Johanson, M.D. Associate Director, Department of Medical Affairs, Genentech, Inc., South San Francisco, California

Eric T. Juengst, B.S., M.A., Ph.D. Adjunct Assistant Professor, Division of Medical Ethics, Department of Medicine, University of California at San Francisco School of Medicine, San Francisco, California

Selna L. Kaplan, M.D., Ph.D. Director, Pediatric Endocrine Unit, Department of Pediatrics, University of California at San Francisco School of Medicine, San Francisco, California

Jack L. Kostyo, Ph.D. Professor, Department of Physiology, University of Michigan Medical School, Ann Arbor, Michigan

Barbara M. Lippe, M.D. Professor, Department of Pediatrics, University of California at Los Angeles School of Medicine, Los Angeles, California

P. Kay Lund, Ph.D. Assistant Professor, Department of Physiology, University of North Carolina School of Medicine, Chapel Hill, North Carolina

James Manson, B.Sc., F.R.C.S.* Research Fellow, Department of Surgery, Harvard Medical School, and Brigham and Women's Hospital, Boston, Massachusetts

---

Current affiliation
*Registrar, Department of Surgery, University Hospital of South Manchester, Manchester, England

Douglas L. Nelson, M.D.*   Assistant Professor, Department of Dermatology, University of Virginia School of Medicine, Charlottesville, Virginia

John S. Parks, M.D., Ph.D.   Professor, Department of Pediatrics, Emory University School of Medicine, Atlanta, Georgia

Alan D. Rogol, M.D., Ph.D.   Professor, Departments of Pediatrics and Pharmacology, University of Virginia School of Medicine, Charlottesville, Virginia

Ron G. Rosenfeld, M.D.   Associate Professor, Department of Pediatrics, Stanford University School of Medicine, Stanford, California

John Savory, Ph.D.   Professor of Pathology and Biochemistry and Director of Clinical Chemistry and Toxicology Laboratories, Department of Pathology, University of Virginia School of Medicine, Charlottesville, Virginia

Barry M. Sherman, M.D.   Director, Department of Clinical Research, Genentech, Inc., South San Francisco, California

Jean Smal, Ph.D.   Postdoctoral Research Fellow, Department of Diabetes, Endocrinology and Metabolism, City of Hope National Medical Center, Duarte, California

Brian Stabler, Ph.D.   Associate Professor of Psychology, Departments of Psychiatry and Pediatrics, University of North Carolina School of Medicine, Chapel Hill, North Carolina

Elizabeth Sutphen, M.P.H., D.Sc.†   Research Associate, Department of Pediatrics, University of Virginia School of Medicine, Charlottesville, Virginia

Michael O. Thorner, M.B., B.S., F.R.C.P.   Professor of Medicine, Department of Internal Medicine, University of Virginia School of Medicine, Charlottesville, Virginia

---

Current affiliation
*Private practice, Newport News, Virginia
†Senior Analyst, Science and Technology Division, U.S. Army Foreign Science and Technology Center, Charlottesville, Virginia

Louis E. Underwood, M.D.   Professor, Department of Pediatrics, University of North Carolina School of Medicine, Chapel Hill, North Carolina

Judson J. Van Wyk, M.D., Sc.D.(hon.)   Kenan Professor of Pediatrics, Department of Pediatrics, University of North Carolina School of Medicine, Chapel Hill, North Carolina

Ashok N. Vaswani, M.D.   Associate Director of Endocrinology and Metabolism, Department of Medicine, Winthrop–University Hospital, Mineola, New York

Douglas W. Wilmore, M.D.*   Professor, Department of Surgery, Harvard Medical School and Brigham and Women's Hospital, Boston, Massachusetts

---

Current affiliation
*Professor, Department of Surgery, Brigham and Women's Hospital, Boston, Massachusetts

HUMAN GROWTH HORMONE

1

Receptors and Biological Effects of Human Growth Hormone and Its Natural 20,000-Molecular-Weight Variant

PIERRE DE MEYTS
and JEAN SMAL

City of Hope
National Medical Center
Duarte, California

M. MAPOKO ILONDO

University of Leuven
School of Medicine
Leuven, Belgium

JEAN CLOSSET
and GEORGES HENNEN

University of Liege
Liege, Belgium

Understanding of the mode of action of growth hormone and characterization of its receptors have been hampered by several factors (1–3). First, growth hormone in pituitary extracts and in plasma is heterogeneous (4–6), the major component being a single-chain peptide of 191 amino acids with a molecular weight of 22,000 daltons (22-KD

1

hGH). The principal variant is 20-KD hGH, which appears to be a direct product of the same hGH N gene, with a deletion resulting from alternative mRNA splicing (7,8). Dimeric, aggregated, and proteolytically degraded forms are also present. In addition to the N gene coding for the main 22- and 20-KD hGH, a variant hGH-V gene, which is not expressed at the pituitary level, codes in vitro for a 191 residue polypeptide of which 13 residues differ from native hGH (9,10). Recently a form of hGH produced by the human placenta and present in maternal serum also has been described. This placental hGH acts as a complete agonist of 22-KD hGH for binding to hepatic GH receptors (11). Finally, some of the higher molecular weight hGH circulating in plasma may result from binding to a plasma protein (12). It is not clear whether these various forms of hGH share the same pattern of biological actions.

The second factor for complicating studies of hGH action is that hGH exerts a variety of biological effects (1–3), its major ones being stimulation of skeletal and somatic growth (increased chondrogenesis and linear skeletal growth, increased protein synthesis, increased cell proliferation). Study of the growth-promoting properties of hGH is complex, because the properties cannot be reproduced directly in vitro. This led to the concept that these effects are indirect, being mediated through a group of substances called somatomedins (13). Recently, however, some direct effects of hGH on DNA synthesis, cell proliferation, and differentiation have been observed in a few cell types (2), and one such effect is now used as a sensitive bioassay (14). Besides its promotion of growth, hGH exerts long-term anti-insulin effects on carbohydrate metabolism and lipolytic effects on fat. Paradoxically, short-term transient insulinlike effects are also seen in vitro and in vivo in models devoid of GH (1,2,15,16). The complex effects of hGH on carbohydrate and lipid metabolism have been reviewed recently by Davidson (17).

Third, growth hormone interferes effectively in various in vivo and in vitro bioassays for lactogens because of its structural similarities with lactogenic hormones such as human prolactin and choriosomatomammotropin (18–21). Lactogenic hormones, in contrast, usually are weak promoters of growth (3,22). This dual pattern of activities is confusing, however, because it depends on the species from which the hormone is derived and on the species tested for the effect (23). Generally, primate growth hormones are strong growth and lactogen agonists in both primates and nonprimates (24–26), whereas nonprimate growth hormones have negligible lactogenic and growth-promoting effects in primates (23–25).

Since the description of the first radioreceptor assay for hGH (27), various in vitro systems have been used to characterize growth hormone receptors, and attempts have been made to link these to the actions of growth hormone. Hughes and colleagues (28,29) conclude from published evidence that different classes of receptors may be associated with the various actions of GH. We concur with this conclusion and will present our recent work on hGH binding sites (and especially their interaction with both 22- and 20-KD hGH) in various in vitro systems, focusing especially on IM-9 human lymphocytes and isolated rat adipocytes.

I. PREPARATION OF RADIOIODINATED ^{125}I-hGH

Iodogen Method

In our studies comparing 22- and 20-KD hGH binding (30–33), both tracers as well as ovine prolactin and bovine somatotropin were labeled in the Liege laboratory by the iodogen method of Fraker and Speck (34). Iodogen (20 μg) and Na^{125}I (1 mCi) were used to label 15 μg of hGH dissolved in 20 μl of 0.5 M phosphate buffer adjusted to pH 7.4 for 5 minutes at room temperature. A similar procedure was used for the labeling of the human 20-KD variant (Figure 1) except that 22 μg of the protein was labeled in 10 minutes. Both tracers were purifed on an Ultrogel Aca 54 column according to the conditions described in Figure 1.

Reverse-Phase High-Performance Liquid Chromatography

We also have used ^{125}I-hGH labeled by the stoichiometric modification (35) of the chloramine-T method (36). These labeled peptides have specific activities of 50–80 μCi/μg and are purified on a 90 ×

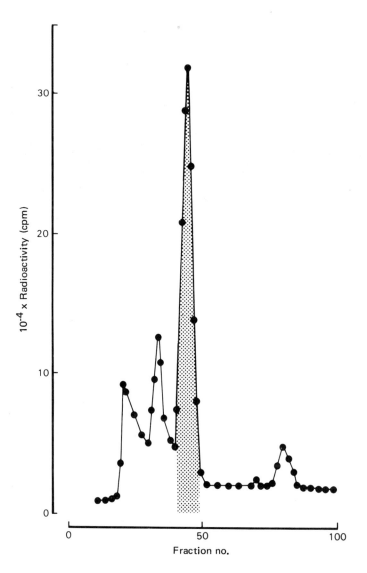

Figure 1. Chromatography of ^{125}I-labeled 20-KD hGH on Ultrogel ACA 54. The column (1 × 100 cm) was equilibrated in a 0.05 *M* sodium phosphate buffer, pH 7.4, containing 0.1% bovine serum albumin. Fraction volumes were 1 ml; a sample of 1 mCi was applied in 1 ml. The shaded area contains the ^{125}I-labeled 20,000 dalton variant monomer. (From Ref. 30.)

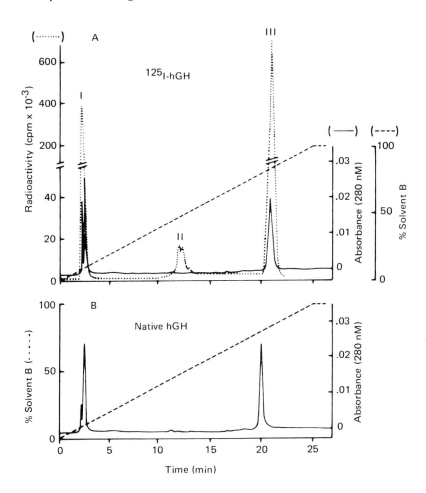

Figure 2. RP-HPLC of ¹²⁵I-hGH (A) and native hGH (B). Column: C18 Synchropak RP-P (250 × 4.1 mm ID). Mobile phase: solvent A, water + TFA 0.1%; solvent B, acetonitrile + TFA 0.1%; linear gradient (----); flow rate, 1 ml/minute; fraction volume 0.3 ml; chart speed, 1 cm/min. UV absorbance at 280 nm (—); radioactivity, cpm/fraction (·····). A: injection, 20 μl of the crude iodinated mixture. B: injection, 25 μg of hGH in 20 μl water. (From Ref. 37.)

1.5 cm Sephadex G-100 column equilibrated and eluted with 0.03 *M* phosphate buffer containing 1 mg/ml of human serum albumin, pH 7.4.

More recently (37) we have purified tracer using a quick and efficient RP-HPLC method, similar to that used at Genentech for characterization of biosynthetic hGH (38). RP-HPLC was conducted at room temperature using a C-18 SynChropak RP-P (Altech, USA) with dimensions of 250 × 4.1 mm. The mobile phase consisted of two solvents. Solvent A was a mixture of water and TFA 0.1% and solvent B a mixture of acetonitrile and TFA 0.1%. A linear gradient was run from 0 to 100% solvent B within 30 minutes. The flow rate was 1 ml/minute. A typical profile is seen in Figure 2. Both methods gave excellent results, with 85% of tracer binding to an excess of receptors (sometimes requiring a two-step assay, ref. 37). It should also be noted that the radioiodinated hormones purified by the iodogen method had been subjected to an HPLC purification step before labeling (31).

II. IM-9 LYMPHOCYTE HUMAN GROWTH HORMONE RECEPTORS: BINDING KINETICS, INTERNALIZATION, AND DOWNREGULATION

The IM-9 human cultured lymphocyte appears at first sight to be a simple system for studying human somatogenic receptors. These cells bear a single population of sites with a very narrow specificity, that of a receptor for the growth-promoting effects of primate growth hormones (22,31,39). Indeed, only hGH (but not nonprimate GHs and lactogenic hormones) is capable of competing significantly for ^{125}I-hGH binding to these cells. This contrasts with the strong reactivity of bovine GH for rabbit liver receptors (39) and of several nonprimate GHs for rat adipocyte receptors (see below). Figures 3 and 4 illustrate the specificity of IM-9 lymphocyte hGH receptors.

IM-9 cells are readily accessible to biochemical manipulations, but unfortunately they have no demonstrable biological response to hGH (apart from the induction of receptor downregulation). Therefore, the IM-9 system is not useful for studying the postreceptor steps in the

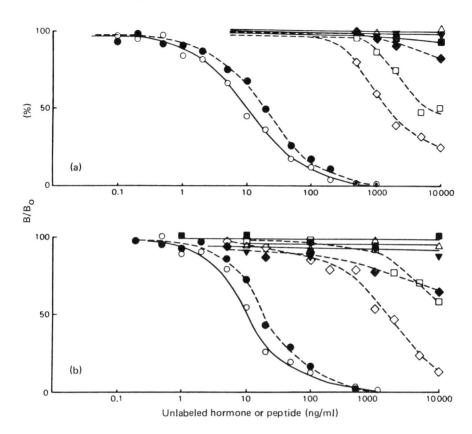

Figure 3. Competition of various animal growth hormones and fragments for ^{125}I-22- (top) and 20-KD (bottom) hGH binding to IM-9 lymphocytes. The tracer used for the studies in the top panel is ^{125}I-22,000-Mr-GH ($\sim$7500 cpm). For studies in the bottom panel, the tracer is ^{125}I-20,000-Mr-GH ($\sim$7500 cpm). IM-9 lymphocytes (2×10^7 cells/ml) were incubated for 10 hours at 30°C with each of the tracers plus increasing concentrations (0.1–10,000 ng/ml) of unlabeled 22,000-Mr-GH (○), 20,000-Mr-GH (●), pGH (▼), bGH (■), eGH (◆), 1–134 hGH peptide (◇), 141–191 hGH peptide (□), or 32–46 hGH peptide (△). B/B_0 in the specific radioactivity bound in the absence of unlabeled hormone. (From Ref. 31.)

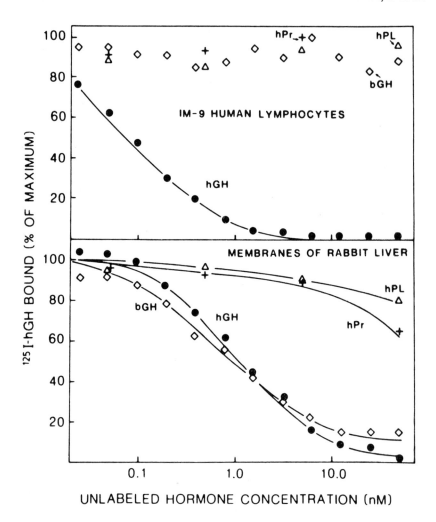

Figure 4.   Competition of human and bovine GH, human prolactin, and placental lactogen for [125]I-22-KD hGH binding to IM-9 lymphocytes (top) and pregnant rabbit liver membranes (bottom). (From Ref. 39.)

somatogenic effects of hGH. The system, however, has proved useful for characterizing receptor binding kinetics (40), downregulation by physiological concentrations of hGH (41), and internalization of hGH-receptor complexes (40,42).

While the existence of linear Scatchard plots for ^{125}I-hGH binding to IM-9 lymphocytes suggested simple mass-action kinetics, the kinetics proved to be extremely complex. Association of ^{125}I-hGH to IM-9 cells proceeds slowly and fails to reach a steady state before 8–10 hours. Dissociation is not first order; instead, a slow component increases in a time- and temperature-dependent manner until binding becomes irreversible (for review, see ref. 40).

The apparent number of hGH binding sites measured in saturation experiments (Scatchard plots) decreases monoexponentially with time of incubation (40). Two separate mechanisms have been postulated to account for the slow component of ^{125}I-hGH dissociation. First, at the level of the receptor there may be a time-dependent generation of a higher-affinity binding state because of a slow conformational change of the receptor (42,43). Second, at the level of the cell, hormone-receptor complexes could be sequestered in a compartment inaccessible to standard dissociation procedures (44,45), for example, by receptor-mediated endocytosis (42). Kinetic studies alone cannot distinguish between these two types of mechanism.

To resolve this issue, we applied the technique of intracellular potassium depletion of Larkin et al. (40,46) to IM-9 lymphocytes. Potassium depletion inhibits coated-pit formation and ligand internalization in some cell lines. IM-9 cells incubated in K$^+$-free buffer after a hypotonic shock lost their K$^+$ rapidly. This was stabilized at ±50% of control by incubation in K$^+$-free binding assay buffer. In K$^+$-depleted cells, the hGH dissociation kinetics became monoexponential (Figure 5) and, in contrast with control cells, was compatible with the equilibrium constant derived from saturation and association data using a simple model. The loss of hGH receptors during competition studies was abolished by K$^+$ depletion (Figure 6), and the downregulation by unlabeled hGH was decreased by 80%. In contrast, insulin receptor kinetics remained unchanged (non-first order) in the K$^+$-depleted cells; the negative cooperativity and the downregulation (60%) were identical to those of control cells. Quantitative electron microscopic autoradi-

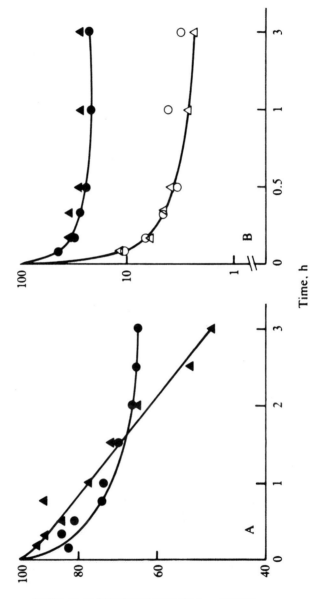

Time, h

ography showed a decrease of $\pm 50\%$ in the fraction of ^{125}I-labeled hGH that was internalized, and the number of visible coated pits in the membrane was reduced by 80%. In IM-9 cells, therefore, association with coated pits and endocytosis appears to play a major role in the kinetics of hGH binding and in the downregulation of its receptors. Because the extent of hGH internalization is smaller than the irreversible binding, it appears that hGH bound to receptors associated with coat pits on the surface is already undissociable.

Figure 5.   Dissociation of bound ^{125}I-hGH (A) and ^{125}I-insulin (B) from control and potassium-depleted IM-9 lymphocytes. (A) Control (●) or K$^+$-depleted (▲) cells (6×10^7/ml) were incubated at 30°C with 80 pM ^{125}I-hGH for 90 minutes. The incubation mixture was then centrifuged at 4°C ($1000 \times$ g for 5 minutes), and the supernatant was replaced by an equal volume of the appropriate assay buffer at 30°C. Duplicate 50-μl aliquots were removed immediately and layered on an equal volume of buffer at 4°C in plastic Microfuge tubes. These tubes were centrifuged immediately. The radioactivity in the cell pellet (22% of total in control cells and 12% of total in K$^+$-depleted cells) represents the amount of ^{125}I-hGH bound at time zero of dissociation. Other 50-μl aliquots were added in triplicate to a series of tubes containing 2.45 ml of assay buffer at 30°C. Sets of tubes were centrifuged at 4°C at each time interval, and the supernatant was discarded. The radioactivity of the cell pellet is expressed as a percentage of the ^{125}I-hGH bound at time zero. (B) Control (●, ○), or K$^+$-depleted (▲, △) cells (5×10^7/ml) were incubated for 60 minutes with 35 pM ^{125}I-insulin at 15°C. At the end of the association, the incubation mixture was processed as in A. Aliquots (50 μl) were added to two series of tubes containing 1.95 ml of either hormone-free buffer, with (●) or without (▲) K$^+$, or assay buffer with (○) or without (△) K$^+$ to which 170 nM unlabeled insulin had been added. The dissociation was assayed as described for A. The amount of tracer bound is expressed as a percentage of the ^{125}I-insulin bound at time zero (80% of total). (From Ref. 40.)

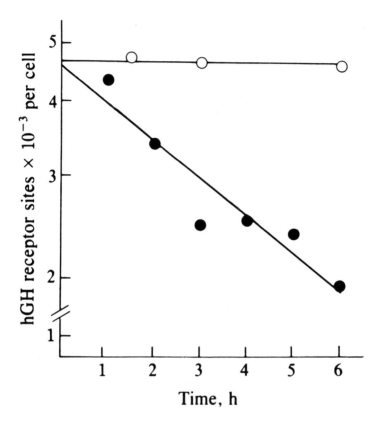

Figure 6. Decrease in the hGH receptor concentration during simultaneous incubation with labeled and unlabeled hGH in normal and potassium-depleted IM-9 lymphocytes. Control (●) or K^+-depleted (○) cells (10^7 in 0.5 ml) were incubated at 30°C with 40 pM ^{125}I-hGH together with increasing concentrations of unlabeled hGH (0–50 nM) for 1–6 hours. The total binding capacity (Ro) was calculated by computer curve fitting of the data and is represented as a function of the duration of incubation. (From Ref. 40.)

III. BINDING AFFINITY OF 22- AND 20-KILODALTON HUMAN GROWTH HORMONE IN IM-9 LYMPHOCYTES AND OTHER "SOMATOGENIC" RECEPTOR SYSTEMS

We recently studied (30–33,47) the biochemical properties of the 20-KD hGH variant of hGH and attempted to identify the receptor-mediated pathways that might explain the discrepancy reported between the growth-promoting and the direct metabolic effects of the variant. Whereas the growth-promoting and lactogenic activities of the 20- and 22-KD forms of hGH are quantitatively similar in various bioassays after in vivo administration (30,48–50), controversy has arisen regarding their effects on glucose metabolism. The 20-KD variant was reported initially (51) to lack the diabetogenic activities of hGH (induction of hyperglycemia and glucose intolerance in dogs), but recent studies show that recombinant 20-KD hGH has essentially the same diabetogenic activity as 22-KD hGH in ob/ob mice (52) and dogs (53). Similarly, early studies suggested that 20-KD hGH lacked the acute insulinlike actions of native-hGH (54). Later, however, recombinant 20-KD hGH was shown to have weak (20%) in vitro insulinlike activity in epididymal adipose tissue of hypophysectomized rats (52).

We recently compared the potency of native and 20-KD hGH in various receptor preparations (30–33). The preparations of 20- and 22-KD hGH were purified in the Liege laboratory, and they were of high quality in terms of cross-contamination, biological activity, and monomeric nature. We first studied pregnant rabbit liver membranes, which contain both somatogenic and lactogenic receptors (30). The data obtained suggested that 20-KD hGH was bound to the same receptors as 22-KD hGH, with a good affinity ($\pm$50%) relative to 22-KD hGH for the somatogenic receptor and an even higher affinity for the lactogenic receptor.

Previous investigations of this problem had yielded a confusing picture. Sigel et al. (55) reported that 20-KD hGH was weak in competing with [125]I-22-KD hGH binding to receptors from pregnant rabbit liver (20-KD hGH = 8–20% of 22-KD hGH), normal female rat liver

(20-KD hGH = 3–12%), and lactating rabbit mammary glands (22–53%). They suggested that 20- and 22-KD hGH may have separate receptors, but no attempt was made to separate somatogenic and lactogenic receptors and labeled 20-KD hGH was not used as a tracer.

Using pregnant rabbit and adult female rat liver, Wohnlich and Moore (56) reported weak competition of 20-KD hGH (6–13% in rabbit, 3% in rat). Using a 20-KD hGH tracer, they observed poor binding by membranes and sixfold weaker binding of ^{125}I-20-KD hGH than ^{125}I-22-KD hGH using pregnant rabbit liver receptors. In the latter system, however, unlabeled 20-KD hGH competed better than 22-KD hGH. From these confusing data, they concluded that the binding properties of 20-KD hGH were significantly altered compared to that of 22-KD hGH.

Finally, Hughes et al. (57) probed both somatogenic and lactogenic receptors of nonpregnant rabbit and pregnant rat liver membranes. They found that the somatogenic receptors in rat liver bind 20-KD hGH with an affinity only slightly lower than that for 22-KD hGH, and that two distinct subsets of somatogenic receptors are present in the rabbit. One small subset of these binds 20-KD hGH with high affinity.

Thus definitive conclusions on the structure-activity of hGH liver receptors are elusive, given the diversity of species used by various investigators, the differing physiological states of the animals (age, male vs. female, pregnant vs. nonpregnant), and the heterogeneity of receptor subpopulations (lactogenic vs. somatogenic, one or several subsets of the latter). Moreover, various tracers and competing hormones have not been used systematically to discriminate between possible receptor subtypes. This is why in a second step we chose to use the simpler IM-9 cultured lymphocyte system (31). We showed that this receptor recognizes the 20-KD variant with 50–60% of the affinity for 20-KD hGH (Figure 7, bottom). These data were consistent with the high potency of 20-KD hGH in bioassays for growth-promoting and lactogenic effects. From all of our liver and IM-9 receptor data as well as the in vivo bioassay results, we conclude that 20-KD hGH is a relatively potent agonist of 22-KD hGH for the somatogenic and lactogenic receptors of humans, rats, and rabbits.

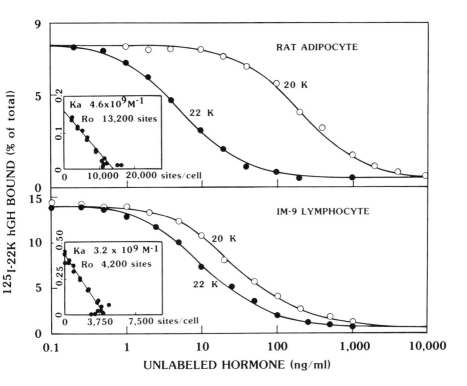

Figure 7. Competition of 22- and 20-KD hGH for [125]I-22-KD hGH binding to rat adipocytes (top) and IM-9 lymphocytes (bottom). In the top panel, 1.6 × 10[6] rat adipocytes/ml were incubated with [125]I-22-KD hGH (40 pM) for 75 minutes at 37°C. In the bottom panel, 20 × 10[6] lymphocytes/ml were incubated with [125]I-22-KD hGH (40 pM) for 10 hours at 30°C. In both systems, unlabeled 22- or 20-KD hGH in amounts ranging from 0.1 to 10,000 ng/ml was added. The fraction of tracer bound is plotted as a function of the concentration of competing hGH. *Insets:* Scatchard plots of the 22-KD competition data. The solid line is drawn according to the computer-filled parameters. The apparent affinity constant is Ka and the binding capacity is Ro. (From Ref. 32.)

IV. BINDING AFFINITY AND BIOLOGICAL EFFECTS OF 22- AND 20-KILODALTON HUMAN GROWTH HORMONES IN ISOLATED RAT ADIPOCYTES

In contrast with our findings in IM-9 lymphocytes, pregnant rabbit liver, and mammary glands, we found (32) that 20-KD hGH has a weak affinity (3%) for the hGH receptor of freshly isolated rat adipocytes (Figure 7, top). This low potency was intrinsic to the 20-KD hGH, because contamination with 22-KD hGH was ≤0.4% as measured by a radioimmunoassay using a specific monoclonal antibody. The lower relative affinity of the 20-KD hGH for rat adipocyte receptors could be caused by species differences rather than tissue specificity. We do not believe that this is the case, because Hughes et al. (57) reported that the affinity of the 20-KD hGH for rat liver receptors is only slightly lower than that of 22-KD hGH, and 20-KD hGH has a growth-promoting activity similar to that of 22-KD hGH in the rat tibia test (48,49). Other specificity differences between the rat adipocyte receptor and the IM-9 lymphocyte receptor (e.g., cross-reactivity of bovine, porcine, rat, and mouse GH in the adipocyte but not in the IM-9 system; ref. 58) are more difficult to ascribe to the tissue rather than to the species. To conclude, the relative affinity of 20-KD hGH for the human IM-9 lymphocyte receptor is consistent with its potent growth-promoting activity, especially since the lower metabolic clearance rate in vivo of 20-KD hGH (59) would compensate for the slight decrease in receptor binding. Conversely, the very low relative binding affinity of 20-KD hGH for the rat adipocyte receptor is consistent with its reported low insulinlike activity. Thus the receptors for hGH on various target cells appear to be different, explaining why the 20-KD variant has different relative biological potency at different sites of action.

We recently were able to establish direct correlations between binding and insulinlike effects on 22- and 20-KD hGH in rat adipocytes (60). We compared the insulinlike effects of 22- and 20-KD hGH using a sensitive assay based on the stimulation of lipogenesis (61). Because hGH did not stimulate lipogenesis in freshly isolated adipocytes from normal animals, we studied adipocytes from hypophysectomized (hypox) rats and from normal rats. We studied adipocytes that were preincubated in vitro without hGH. The binding characteristics in the three models (normal fresh, hypox, normal preincubated) were similar: the affinity constant of 22-KD hGH = $5 \times 10^9 \, M^{-1}$, the receptor number was 10,000–15,000 sites/cell, the potency of 20-KD hGH was 3% that of 22-KD hGH. In fat cells from hypox rats, the highest dose of hGH stimulated the incorporation of D-(3-^{3}H) glucose into lipids by 30% maximally; the dose-response curve for 20-KD hGH was shifted to the right but the model was too insensitive for a precise potency estimate. In fat cells from normal rats, stimulation of lipogenesis by hGH increased with time of preincubation; at 5 hours, the maximal stimulation was 200–250%. The curve for 20-KD hGH had the same maximum, but a relative potency of only 2–6% that of 22-KD hGH. Maximum stimulation of lipogenesis by insulin was six to seven times higher than with hGH, and the half maximal effect dose was $4 \times 10^{-11} \, M$ for insulin vs. $1.5 \times 10^{-9} \, M$ for 22-KD hGH. When combined, nonmaximal doses of hGH and insulin were 25% more than strictly additive. An intermediate dose of insulin (0.1 ng/ml) was 25% more than additive to a maximal dose of hGH (1000 ng/ml). In contrast, the combined stimulation by maximally effective doses of hGH and insulin was indentical to that by insulin alone (60). These studies will be reported in full elsewhere (33).

In conclusion, preincubated rat adipocytes are a sensitive model for investigating the structure–activity relationships of the direct effects of hGH. The 20-KD variant is only 3% as potent as 22-KD hGH, for binding and bioactivity, confirming that the adipocyte receptor is different from that promoting the growth effects. The additivity data suggest that hGH shares only a subset of the metabolic pathways activated by insulin, a finding that will be useful in deciphering the mode of action of insulin as well as that of hGH (60). Figure 8 is a schematic model of our concept of insulin and hGH actions on lipogenesis.

Since phorbol esters also activate lipogenesis in rat adipocytes (62,63) and, like hGH, have a smaller maximal effect than insulin, hGH might share a kinase-C pathway of insulin action in adipocytes. Nevertheless, data concerning involvement of kinase-C in insulin actions in adipocytes are still conflicting (64,65). We are now attempting to dissect the metabolic steps shared by insulin and hGH in rat adipocytes more precisely (66).

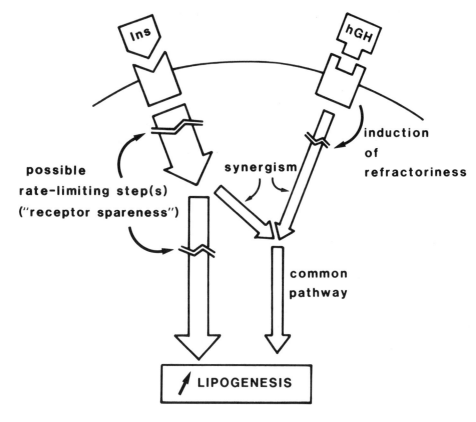

Figure 8. Our hypothesis of separate and common pathways of insulin and hGH actions on lipogenesis in isolated rat adipocytes.

REFERENCES

1. Merimee TJ. Growth hormone: Secretion and action. In Endocrinology, Vol. 1, DeGroot LJ, ed. Grune and Stratton, New York, 1979, pp. 123–132.

2. Isaksson OGP, Eden S, Jansson JO. Mode of action of pituitary growth hormone on target cells. Ann. Rev. Physiol. 47:483–499, 1985.

3. Underwood LE, Van Wyk JJ. Normal and aberrant growth. In Williams Textbook of Endocrinology, 7th ed., Wilson JD, Foster DW, eds., Saunders, Philadelphia, 1985, pp. 155–205.

4. Lewis UJ, Singh RNP, Tutwiler GF, Sigel MB, Vanderlaan EF, Vanderlaan WP. Human growth hormone: A complex of proteins. Rec. Prog. Horm. Res. 36:477–508, 1980.

5. Lewis UJ. Heterogeneity of growth hormone in the pituitary gland. In Endocrinology, Proceedings of the 7th International Congress on Endocrinology, Labrie F, Proulx L, eds., Excerpta Medica, Amsterdam, 1984, pp. 745–748.

6. Baumann G. Heterogeneity of growth hormone in the circulation. In Endocrinology, Proceedings of the 7th International Congress on Endocrinology, Labrie F, Proulx L, eds., Excerpta Medica, Amsterdam, 1984, pp. 749–752.

7. Wallis M. Growth hormone: Deletions in the protein and introns in the gene. Nature 284:512, 1980.

8. De Noto FM, Moore DD, Goodman HM. Human growth hormone DNA sequence and mRNA structure: Possible alternative splicing. Nucleic Acids Res. 9:3719–3730, 1981.

9. Pavlakis GN, Hizuka N, Gorden PL, Seeburg P, Hamer DH. Expression of two human growth hormone genes in monkey cells infected by simian virus 40 recombinants. Proc. Natl. Acad. Sci. USA 78:7398–7402, 1981.

10. Seeburg PH. The human growth hormone gene family: Nucleotide sequences show recent divergence and predict a new polypeptide hormone. DNA 1:239–249, 1982.

11. Hennen G, Frankenne F, Closset J, Gomez F, Pirens G, El Khayat N. A human placental GH: Increasing levels during second half of pregnancy with pituitary GH suppression as revealed by monoclonal antibody. Int. J. Fert. 30:27–33, 1985.

12. Baumann G, Stolar MW, Amburn K, Barsano CP, DeVries BC. A specific growth hormone-binding protein in human plasma: Initial characterization. J. Clin. Endocrinol. Metab. 62:134–141, 1986.

13. Daughaday WH, Hall K, Raben MS, Salmon WD, Van Den Brande JL, Van Wyk JJ. Somatomedin: Proposed designation for sulphation factor. Nature 235:107, 1972.

14. Rayhel ES, Albright JF, Shenk BA, Hughes JP. Stimulation of NB2 cell growth by interleukin 2 and human growth hormone. The Endocrine Society, 68th Annual Meeting, Abstract 750, 1986, p. 218.

15. Goodman HM. Separation of early and late responses of adipose tissue to growth hormone. Endocrinology 109:120–129, 1981.

16. Carter-Su C, Rosza F. Growth hormone causes rapid and transitory stimulation of glucose transport in rat adipocytes. The Endocrine Society, 68th Annual Meeting, Abstract 373, 1986, p. 124.

17. Davidson MB. Effect of growth hormone on carbohydrate and lipid metabolism: A review. In Acromegaly Centennial Symposium, Robbins R, Melmed S, eds. Plenum, New York. (in press)

18. Bangham DR, Gaines Das RE, Schulster D. The international standard for human growth hormone for bioassay. Calibration and characterization by international collaborative study. Mol. Cell. Endocrinol. 42: 269–282, 1985.

19. Lyons WR, Li CH, Johnson RE. The hormonal control of mammary growth and lactation. Rec. Prog. Horm. Res. 14:219–254, 1958.

20. Rimoin DL, Holzman GB, Merimee TJ. Lactation in the absence of human growth hormone. J. Clin. Endocrinol. Metab. 28:1183–1188, 1968.

21. Frantz AG, Wilson JD. Endocrine disorders of the breast. In Williams Textbook of Endocrinology, Wilson JD, Foster DW, eds., Saunders, Philadelphia, 1985, pp. 402–421.

22. Lesniak MA, Gorden P, Roth J. Reactivity of non-primate growth hormones and prolactins with human growth hormone receptors on cultured human lymphocytes. J. Clin. Endocrinol. Metab. 44:838–849, 1977.

23. Bewley TA, Li CH. The chemistry of human pituitary growth hormone. In Advances in Enzymology, vol. 42, Meister A, ed., Wiley, New York, 1975, pp. 73–166.

24. Knobil E, Wolf RC, Greep RO. Some physiologic effects of primate pituitary growth hormone preparations in the hypophysectomized Rhesus monkey. J. Clin. Endocrinol. Metab. 16:916, 1956.

25. Knobil E, Greep RO. The physiology of growth hormone with particular reference to its action in the Rhesus monkey and the "species specificity" problem. Rec. Prog. Horm. Res. 15:1–36, 1959.

26. Peckham WD, Hotchkiss J, Knobil E, Nicoll CS. Prolactin activity of homogeneous primate growth hormone preparations. Endocrinology 82: 1247–1248, 1968.

27. Lesniak MA, Roth J, Gorden P, Gavin JR III. Human growth hormone radioreceptor assay using cultured human lymphocytes. Nature (New Biol.) 241:20–21, 1973.

28. Hughes JP, Elsholtz HP, Friesen HG. Growth hormone and prolactin receptors. In Polypeptide Hormone Receptors, Posner BI, ed., Marcel Dekker, New York, 1985, pp. 157–199.

29. Hughes JP, Friesen HG. The nature and regulation of the receptors for pituitary growth hormone. Ann. Rev. Physiol. 47:469–482, 1985.

30. Closset J, Smal J, Gomez F, Hennen G. Purification of the 22000- and 20000-mol. wt. forms of human somatotropin and characterization of their binding to liver and mammary binding sites. Biochem. J. 214: 885–892, 1983.

31. Smal J, Closset J, Hennen G, De Meyts P. Receptor-binding and down-regulatory properties of 22000-Mr human growth hormone and its natural 20000-Mr variant on IM-9 human lymphocytes. Biochem. J. 225: 283–289, 1985.

32. Smal J, Closset J, Hennen G, De Meyts P. The receptor binding properties of the 20K variant of human growth hormone explain its discrepant insulin-like and growth promoting activities. Biochem. Biophys. Res. Commun. 134:159–165, 1986.

33. Smal J, Closset J, Hennen G, De Meyts P. Receptor binding properties and insulin-like effects of human growth hormone and its 20K variant in rat adipocytes. J. Biol. Chem., 1987 (in press).

34. Fraker PJ, Speck JC. Protein and cell membrane iodinations with a sparingly soluble chloroamide, 1,3,4,6-tetrachloro-3α,6α-diphenylglycoluril. Biochem. Biophys. Res. Commun. 80:849–857, 1978.

35. Roth J. Method for assessing immunologic and biologic properties of iodinated peptide hormones. In Methods in Enzymology, vol. 37, O'Malley BW, Hardman JG, eds., Academic Press, New York, 1975, pp. 223–233.

36. Hunter WM, Greenwood FC. Preparation of iodine-131 labeled human growth hormone of high specific activity. Nature 194:495–496, 1962.

37. Ilondo MM, Dehart I, De Meyts P. A rapid method for the preparation of ^{125}I-labeled human growth hormone for receptor studies, using reverse-phase high performance liquid chromatography. Biochem. Biophys. Res. Commun. 134:671–677, 1986.

38. Olson KC, Fenno J, Lin N, Harkins RN, Snicler C, Kohr WH, Ross MJ, Fodge D, Prender G, Stebbing N. Purified human growth hormone from E. coli is biologically active. Nature 293:409–411, 1981.

39. Retegui LA, De Meyts P, Pena C, Masson PL. The same region of human growth hormone is involved in its binding for various receptors. Endocrinology 111:668–676, 1982.

40. Ilondo MM, Courtoy PJ, Geiger D, Carpentie.· JL, Rousseau GG, De Meyts P. Intracellular potassium depletion in IM-9 lymphocytes suppresses the slowly dissociating component of human growth hormone binding and the downregulation of its receptors but does not affect insulin receptors. Proc. Natl. Acad. Sci. USA 83:6460–6464, 1986.

41. Lesniak MA, Roth J. Regulation of receptor concentration by homologous hormone. Effect of human growth hormone on its receptor in IM-9 lymphocytes. J. Biol. Chem. 251:3720–3729, 1976.

42. Barrazone P, Lesniak MA, Gorden P, Van Obberghen E, Carpentier JL, Orci L. Binding, internalization, and lysosomal association of ^{125}I-human growth hormone in cultured human lymphocytes: A quantitative morphological and biochemical study. J. Cell. Biol. 87:360–369, 1981.

43. Donner DB. Interconversion between different states of affinity of the human growth hormone receptor on rat hepatocytes: Effects of fractional site occupancy on receptor availability. Biochemistry 19:3300–3306, 1980.

44. Rosenfeld RG, Hintz RL. Compartmentalization of human growth hormone by cultured human lymphocytes. J. Clin. Endocrinol. Metab. 51:368–375, 1980.

45. Donner DB, Martin DW, Sonenberg M. Accumulation of a slowly dissociable peptide hormone binding component by isolated target cells. Proc. Natl. Acad. Sci. USA 75:672–676, 1978.

46. Larkin JM, Brown MS, Goldstein JL, Anderson RGW. Depletion of intracellular potassium arrests coated pit formation and receptor-mediated endocytosis in fibroblasts. Cell 33:273–285, 1983.

47. Smal J. Etude des proprietes biologiques de l'hormone de croissance humaine et de son variant 20K, Ph.D. diss., Catholic University of Louvain, Belgium, 1986.

48. Lewis UJ, Dunn JT, Bonewald LF, Seavay BK, Vanderlaan WP. A naturally occurring structural variant of human growth hormone. J. Biol. Chem. 253:2679–2687, 1978.

49. Chapman GE, Rogers KM, Brittain T, Bradshaw RA, Bates OJ, Turner C, Cary PD, Crane-Robinson C. The 20,000 molecular weight variant of human growth hormone. Preparation and some physical and chemical properties. J. Biol. Chem. 256:2395–2401, 1981.

50. Spencer EM, Lewis LJ, Lewis UJ. Somatomedin generating activity of the 20,000-dalton variant of human growth hormone. Endocrinology 109:1301–1302, 1981.

51. Lewis UJ, Singh RNP, Tutwiler GF. Hyperglycemic activity of the 20,000-dalton variant of human growth hormone. Endocrinol. Res. Commun. 8:155–164, 1981.

52. Kostyo JL, Cameron CM, Olson KC, Jones AJS, Pai RC. Biosynthetic 20-kilodalton methionyl-human growth hormone has diabetogenic and insulin-like activities. Proc. Natl. Acad. Sci. USA 82:4250–4253, 1985.

53. Ader M, Agajanian T, Finegood D, Bergman RN. Recombinant DNA-derived 22K- and 20K-human growth hormone (hGH) generate equivalent diabetogenic effects during chronic infusion in dogs. Endocrinology 120:725–731, 1987.

54. Frigeri LJ, Peterson SM, Lewis UJ. The 20,000-dalton structural variant of human growth hormone: Lack of some early insulin-like effects. Biochem. Biophys. Res. Commun. 91:778–779, 1979.

55. Sigel MB, Thorpe NA, Kobrin MS, Lewis UJ, Vanderlaan WP. Binding characteristics of a biologically active variant of human growth hormone (20K) to growth hormone and lactogen receptors. Endocrinology 108:1600–1603, 1981.

56. Wohnlich L, Moore WB. Binding of a variant of human growth hormone to liver plasma membranes. Horm. Metab. Res. 14:138–141, 1982.

57. Hughes JP, Tokuhiro E, Steven J, Simpson A, Friesen HG. 20K is

bound with high affinity by one rat and one of two rabbit growth hormone receptors. Endocrinology 113:1904–1906, 1983.

58. Gavin JR, Stalman RJ, Tollefsen SE. Growth hormone receptors in isolated rat adipocytes. Endocrinology 110:637–643, 1982.

59. Baumann G, Stolar MW, Buchanan TA. Slow metabolic clearance rate of the 20,000-dalton variant of human growth hormone: Implications for biological activity. Endocrinology 117:1309–1313, 1985.

60. Smal J, Closset J, Hennen G, De Meyts P. Receptor binding and insulin-like effects of 22K human growth hormone and its 20K variant in the rat adipocytes. The Endocrine Society, 68th Annual Meeting, Abstract 365, 1986, p. 122.

61. Moody AJ, Stan MA, Stan M. A simple free fat cell bioassay for insulin. Horm. Metab. Res. 6:12–16, 1974.

62. Skoglund G, Hansson A, Ingelman Sundberg M. Rapid effects of phorbol esters on isolated rat adipocytes. Relationship to the action of protein kinase c. Eur. J. Biochem. 148:407–412, 1985.

63. Van de Werve G, Proietto J, Jeanrenaud B. Tumor-promoting phorbol esters increase basal and inhibit insulin-stimulated lipogenesis in rat adipocytes without decreasing insulin binding. Biochem. J. 225:523–527, 1985.

64. Glynn BP, Colliton JW, McDermott JM, Witter LA. Phorbol esters, but not insulin, promote depletion of cytosolic protein kinase C in rat adipocytes. Biochem. Biophys. Res. Commun. 135:1119–1125, 1986.

65. Cherqui G, Caron M, Wicek D, Lascols O, Capeau J, Picard J. Decreased insulin responsiveness in fat cells rendered protein kinase C-deficient by a treatment with a phorbol ester. Endocrinology 120: 2192–2194, 1987.

66. Smal J, De Meyts P. Role of kinase C in the insulinlike effects of human growth hormone on rat adipocytes. Serono International Symposium on Growth Hormone (abstract), 1987 (in press).

2

Indirect Actions of Growth Hormone

JUDSON J. VAN WYK, SAMUEL J. CASELLA,*
MARY HYNES, and P. KAY LUND
University of North Carolina
School of Medicine
Chapel Hill, North Carolina

A fundamental problem in understanding the mechanisms of growth hormone action is the lack of concordance between its effects in vivo and in vitro. The hypothesis of Salmon and Daughaday that GH exerts its growth-promoting effects indirectly was the result of their efforts to develop a bioassay that possessed sufficient sensitivity to be useful as a clinical test of GH status in man (1). Although the activity of serum in their sulfation factor assay paralleled the GH status of the

*Current affiliation: Johns Hopkins University School of Medicine, Baltimore, Maryland.

This work was supported by USPHS Training Grant AM07129 and Research Grant AM01022 and Career Research Award AM14115.

donor, GH itself was inactive. For this reason they postulated that the growth-promoting actions of GH on the skeleton are indirect and mediated through a factor that is either derived from GH itself or induced in vivo by GH action.

Research on the somatomedins in our laboratory was triggered by Daughaday and Reeder's report in 1966 that administration of GH to hypophysectomized rats stimulated up to an 18-fold increase in thymidine incorporation in cartilage as contrasted with a twofold to threefold increase in sulfate uptake (2). At that time we thought it unlikely that the same signal would serve as the stimulus for both differentiated cell functions and cell replication, and hence we devised a double isotope assay using hypophysectomized rat cartilage to distinguish "thymidine factor" activity from "sulfation factor" activity during the purification of these substances from human blood. Dissociation of the putative differentiating factor from the mitogen failed to occur, however, and the substance that we finally purified was found to stimulate the synthesis of both proteoglycans and DNA in cartilage explants (3). This substance was designated somatomedin-C (Sm-C) by us (4) and insulinlike growth factor I (IGF-I) by Rinderknecht and Humbel (5).

I. CLASSIFICATION OF DIRECT AND INDIRECT EFFECTS OF GROWTH HORMONE

Discussions of which actions of growth hormone in the living body are direct actions and which are indirect actions frequently have been polarized between what might be called the "growth hormone hypothesis of growth hormone action" and the "somatomedin hypothesis of growth hormone action." Such a dichotomy may be overly simplistic, however, since certain observations cannot be satisfactorily explained by either hypothesis. Ellis, Vodian, and Grindeland, for example, reported that a large part of the pituitary-derived growth-promoting activity of rat or human serum, as measured by the tibia test, cannot be accounted for by its content of either immunoreactive GH or somatomedin (6). Also, Golde and co-workers described patients with pituitary tumors and acromegalic features who had neither increased GH nor somatomedin levels in their serum, although serum from these patients was highly active in stimulating the growth of bone marrow cells in culture (7,8).

Such paradoxes may be resolved as we learn more about the biosynthesis and processing of the complex cluster of genes encoding the GH and prolactin family of peptides. For example, we cannot yet exclude the possibility that the variant GH gene may be expressed under certain circumstances, or that alternate gene splicing might lead to currently unrecognized cleavage products with properties that are different from the parent. We now know that about 5–10% of pituitary GH is secreted in the form of the 20-KD variant arising from alternate gene splicing, and Mittra reported that a more drastically cleaved form of GH with a two-chain structure possesses intrinsic, albeit very weak, somatomedinlike activity (9).

There is no intrinsic reason why members of the GH/prolactin family of peptide hormones should require an intermediate for their mitogenic activity, and Isaksson and his colleagues ably summarized the evidence for a direct mitogenic role of GH in many growth processes (10). Golde presented very strong evidence that hGH is a direct mitogen for hematopoietic stem cells (11). Linzer and Nathans found that stimulation of quiescent Balb/c 3T3 cells by serum caused a 15-fold to 20-fold increase in a 1-kb mRNA that encoded a mitogenic peptide that they called proliferin (12). When sequenced, this mitogen proved to be a member of the mouse prolactin family that is normally produced by the placenta in mid-gestation (13)!

Green and co-workers proposed a novel resolution of the controversy between the growth hormone versus somatomedin hypotheses of growth hormone action by his "dual effector model of growth hormone action," in which growth hormone and somatomedin act in tandem at the target site (14). According to this model, GH first stimulates precursor cells to undergo differentiation, and somatomedins then act as mitogens to stimulate clonal growth of the differentiated cells (Figure 1). Although their data were derived from a preadipocyte cell line, Green et al. postulated that their model can just as well be applied to the interactions of GH and somatomedin in cartilage and other tissues. It should be noted, however, that in some tissues the somatomedins are

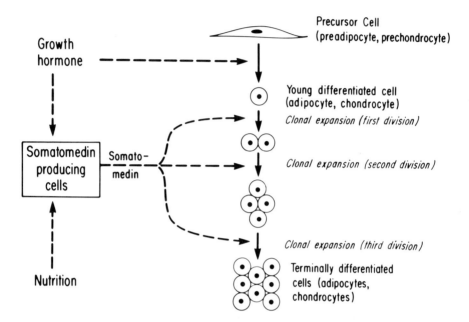

Figure 1. Dual effector theory of GH action as proposed by Green. According to this theory GH acts directly on undifferentiated precursor cells (in this case preadipocytes) to promote differentiation into more mature cells that are capable of clonal expansion into terminally differentiated cells. Growth hormone also stimulates the production of somatomedin in neighboring cells and this, in turn, stimulates the clonal growth of the differentiated cells. (From Ref. 14.)

more active in promoting differentiation than in stimulating cell proliferation, and that even in certain preadipocyte cell lines insulin or insulinlike growth factors are just as essential for differentiation as they are for proliferation (15).

Direct Actions of Growth Hormone

After allowing for certain exceptions as noted, many of the actions of GH in the living body fall into two broad groups: those that are synergistic with cortisol and opposite to the action of insulin, and those that are insulinlike and opposed by the actions of cortisol. As a first

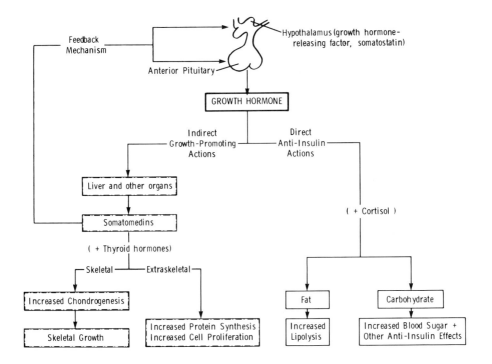

Figure 2. Proposed scheme for characterizing peripheral actions of growth hormone. The direct actions of GH, which are often synergistic with cortisol and antagonistic to insulin, include diabetogenic and lipolytic actions and stimulation of certain hepatic enzymes. Indirect growth-promoting actions, which are insulinlike and antagonized by cortisol, are thought to be mediated through somatomedins. Somatomedins exercise a negative feedback on GH secretion by stimulating somatostatin and by directly antagonizing the effect of GH releasing factor on GH secretion. (From Ref. 16.)

approximation, we have suggested that those actions of GH that are synergized by cortisol are direct effects and require no intermediary (Figure 2) (16). Three examples of such effects follow.

Adipose Tissue

Although GH produces an early insulinlike effect when first administered to hypophysectomized animals, the predominant effect on lipid metabolism is lipolytic with resultant elevation of free fatty acids. Hypopituitary children have stores of ripply fat that melt away with GH administration. The suggestion that an impurity may have been responsible for these lipolytic effects has been dispelled by observing these same effects in GH-deficient children treated with Protropin. Fain and co-workers showed that the lipolytic effect of GH on isolated adipose tissue is not manifested unless glucocorticoids such as dexamethasone are present in the medium (17).

Liver

Growth hormone stimulates many different processes in this organ, some of which are undoubtedly direct and others indirect. Synergism between GH and cortisol has been well documented, however, in the induction of a variety of hepatic enzymes including tyrosine transaminase and tryptophane pyrollase (18) and enzymes of obvious importance in gluconeogenesis such as glucokinase (19). Richman and co-workers showed that cortisol and GH act synergistically on the

Table 1.   Synergistic Effect of Hydrocortisone and Growth Hormone on Induction of Ornithine Decarboxylase in Livers of Hypophysectomized Rats

Treatment[a]	nCi of $^{14}CO_2$/g per 30 min ($\pm$SEM)	No. of rats
Untreated	1.46 ($\pm$0.53)	(12)
hGH 150 μg	13.91 ($\pm$3.16)	(12)
Cortisol 5 mg	88.60 ($\pm$23.76)	(6)
hGH + cortisol	225.88 ($\pm$32.17)	(4)

Measurements of enzymatic activity were made on liver homogenates of hypophysectomized rats 4 hours after the induction of saline, 150 μg of hGH, 5 mg of hydrocortisone, or a combination of the two hormones.
[a]Administered intraperitoneally 4 hours before sacrifice.
Source: Ref. 20.

induction of ornithine decarboxylase in the livers of hypophysectomized rats (20). (See Table 1.)

Carbohydrate Metabolism

The synergistic effect of cortisol and growth hormone in the regulation
of blood sugar was clearly documented in four hypopituitary children
whom we studied during a basal period without therapy, a period with
a 0.5 mg growth hormone daily for several weeks, a period with 25 mg
cortisone daily, and a fourth period in which cortisone and growth
hormone were given concurrently (21). In none of the subjects did
either cortisone alone or GH alone produce much effect on the fasting
blood sugar, and in each case the most significant elevation occurred
when both agents were given together. The higher blood sugar levels
during combined therapy were caused by increased insulin resistance,
since plasma insulin responses to an intravenous glucose tolerance test
were also highest during this period. In each period the four boys were
subjected to a prolonged fast that was terminated by the administration
of glucagon to test their glycogen stores. Neither cortisone nor GH had
much influence on the glycogen stores and both hormones were required to elicit a significant hyperglycemic effect (Figure 3).

Indirect Actions of Growth Hormone

The growth-promoting effects of GH include cell proliferation and
protein synthesis in both skeletal and nonskeletal tissue. In contrast to
the direct actions of GH, many of which are synergistic with cortisol,
the growth-promoting actions of GH are insulinlike and opposed by
cortisol. Indeed, even small excesses of cortisone blunt the effect of
GH in hypopituitary children (22). The evidence is now very strong
that many of the growth-promoting actions of GH are indirect actions
mediated by the somatomedins; indeed, Schoenle et al. showed that
both IGF-I and IGF-II can stimulate growth in hypophysectomized
animals, although the effect of IGF-II is marginal (23,24).

Muscle

Children treated with growth hormone have an increase in both muscle
cell number and cell size (25). This growth is accompanied by a sharp

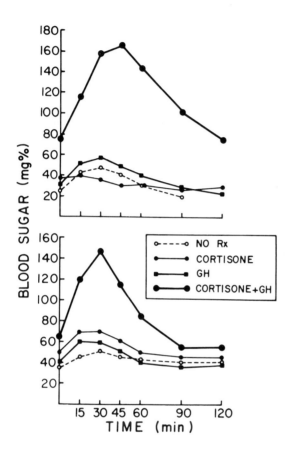

Figure 3. Synergistic effect of cortisone and GH on hepatic glycogen stores. Two boys with severe hypopituitarism were fasted during four different periods as described in the text. Each fast was terminated by the administration of 0.05 mg/kg of aqueous glucagon. Neither cortisone nor GH in the dosages given were by themselves able to improve the glycogen stores significantly over those present in the absence of any treatment. When cortisone and GH were given together, however, their combined effect was dramatic. (From Ref. 21.)

shift to a positive nitrogen balance. In in vitro studies, Florini and co-workers showed that somatomedin stimulates both proliferation of the L6 myoblast cell line and differentiation of myoblasts to myotubes (26).

Cartilage

The special hallmark of GH action is skeletal growth. Growth of the bony skeleton is secondary to primary effects in cartilage, and in the intact animal growth hormone stimulates proliferation of chondrocytes and synthesis of cartilage matrix. In most hands, however, GH has little effect on cartilage growth in vitro, whereas the somatomedins stimulate both proteoglycan and DNA synthesis in cartilage explants or in cultured chrondrocytes.

The somatomedin hypothesis of GH action on skeletal growth was challenged by two studies of Isaksson's group. They injected GH directly into the growth plate of hypophysectomized rabbits and observed significant widening of the epiphyseal plate (27). Although this observation has been repeated in other laboratories, this experiment is difficult to interpret since the dosage of GH was large and could have induced somatomedin production by fibroblasts or other perichondrial cells.

A more direct challenge to the somatomedin hypothesis was the demonstration by Madsen et al. that a noncommercial preparation of GH simulated thymidine incorporation and DNA synthesis in cultured rabbit-ear chondrocytes (28). Although neither our laboratory nor the laboratories of Drs. S. Trippel in Boston or M. Corvol in Paris have been successful in duplicating these results with any commercial preparation of growth hormones (including Protropin), Corvol was able to demonstrate a small increase in ^{3}H-thymidine incorporation with no change in total DNA when she repeated her studies with a preparation of GH purified by methods similar to those used in the Madsen study (personal communication). It thus remains to be determined whether the discrepant results between the various laboratories is attributable to differences in the preparations of GH used in these studies or to some other as yet unidentified variable in experimental design.

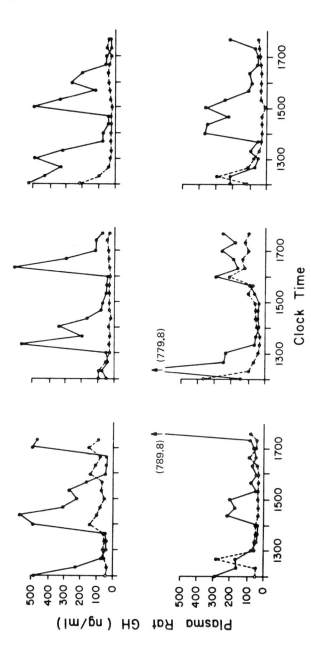

Figure 4. Effect on plasma GH levels of 500 ng of Sm-C injected into rats intraventricularly through a previously implanted catheter. Blood samples were drawn through an indwelling cannula in the right atrium. Each rat was first sampled after a control injection of saline (solid line) 7–10 days previous to the injection of Sm-C (dashed line). The effect of Sm-C was similar to the effect of intraventricular injections of hGH. (From Ref. 29.)

Role of Somatomedins in Growth Hormone Feedback Mechanism

The most compelling evidence that somatomedin plays a crucial physiological role in mediating important actions of GH is the group of observations that implicates somatomedin in the feedback regulation of GH secretion. Abe, Molitch et al. showed that the intraventricular administration of either GH or Sm-C inhibited the episodic spikes of GH in the serum of intact unanesthetized rats (29) (Figure 4). At least two mechanisms appear to account for this inhibitory effect of Sm-C on GH secretion. Berelowitz et al. showed that somatomedin stimulates the production of somatostatin in hypothalamic remnants (30), and Brazeau et al. showed that Sm-C directly inhibits the action of pancreatic GRF on GH release from dispersed pituitary cell cultures (31). Even more convincing was the demonstration by Yamashita and Melmed that Sm-C inhibits the expression of the GH gene in pituitary explants (32). From a teleological standpoint it is difficult to imagine why Sm-C should be involved in the GH feedback loop if it did not mediate critical actions of GH.

II. THE SOMATOMEDIN FAMILY OF PEPTIDE GROWTH FACTORS

Nomenclature and Structure

The confusing nomenclature of the somatomedins has now been substantially clarified by the consensus of most workers that only two peptides account for all, or nearly all, of the biological effects attributed to this "family" of peptide growth factors. Both somatomedins that were isolated from human blood are single-chain peptides that exhibit a high degree of homology with human proinsulin. The basic 70 amino acid residue peptide that we isolated under the name somatomedin C (Sm-C) (4,33,34) proved to be identical to the same peptide that Rinderknecht and Humbel (4) isolated and sequenced under the term insulinlike growth factor I (IGF-I) (Figure 5). By whatever name, Sm-C or IGF-I is more GH dependent and less insulinlike than the neutral peptide insulinlike growth factor II (IGF-II), also described by Rinderknecht and Humbel (35). Multiplication stimulat-

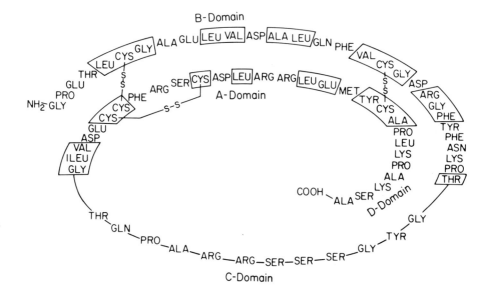

Figure 5. Primary structure of Sm-C/IGF-I. The residues enclosed in boxes in the A and B domains of Sm-C/IGF-I are identical to the amino acids in corresponding positions in human proinsulin. The C-peptides of the somatomedins, however, are much shorter than the C-peptide of proinsulin and exhibit no homology. The D domain is an eight-residue extension at the carboxy terminus that does not exist in proinsulin. The B and A domains of IGF-II are about 70% identical to similar regions in Sm-C/IGF-I. The C domain of IGF-II is composed of eight amino acid residues which are not homologous with the 12 in Sm-C/IGF-I. The D domain of IGF-II is also two residues shorter and not homologous with the D domain of Sm-C/IGF-I. The prohormones for Sm-C/IGF-I and IGF-II have additional E domains that consist of extensions beyond their COOH termini. (From Ref. 16.)

ing factor (MSA) has proven to be the rat counterpart of IGF-II and differs in only five amino acid residues (36).

The Somatomedin Genes

Available evidence suggests that in humans, both of the somatomedins are single copy genes, with the gene for prepro-Sm-C/IGF-I on the short arm of chromosome 12, and the gene for prepro-IGF-II on the short arm of chromosome 11 immediately adjacent to the gene for preproinsulin (37,38). The somatomedin locus on each chromasome is very close to proto-oncogenes of the *c-ras* family.

Sm-C/IGF-I and IGF-II, like many other secreted proteins, are synthesized as larger prohormones with leader sequences of 25 or 24 amino acids at their amino termini, and with longer extensions beyond their carboxy termini. Human liver cDNA libraries have disclosed nucleotide sequences predicting two different Sm-C precursors of 153 and 195 amino acid residues respectively, apparently arising by alternate RNA processing of a single gene (39,40). The liver mRNA for proIGF-II encodes a 185 amino acid residue protein. Thus the prepro forms of the hormones require posttranslational processing to arrive at the mature forms of the hormone. Jansen et al. encountered in a human liver library a cDNA representing a variant form of IGF-II (41). This variant form is also postulated to be the product of alternate splicing of a common RNA precursor.

Interactions of Somatomedins with Their Receptors

In 1971 we reported that somatomedin cross-reacted with insulin in radioreceptor assays (42). Although it was initially believed that this cross-reactivity was fully explained by the structural homology between the peptides themselves, it was subsequently shown that the receptors for insulin and Sm-C/IGF-I are also structurally homologous (43–45). Two distinct somatomedin receptors have been identified, each with a degree of specificity for one of the two major somatomedins: the type I receptor, which has higher affinity for Sm-C/IGF-I, and the type II receptor, which preferentially binds IFG-II. The type I receptor has a heterotetrameric structure similar to that of the insulin receptor, whereas the type II receptor is physically different from either the type I or the insulin receptor, it lacks tyrosine kinase activity, and its function is currently not known (46,47). The structure and relative affinities of these receptors are summarized in Table 2.

Recent evidence from our laboratory points to yet another type of membrane binding site for IGF-II that is immunologically different from the Sm-C/IGF-I binding site on the type I receptor. Casella found that in human placental membranes ^{125}I-IGF-II binds to both 130K and 260K binding sites (type I and type II receptors), but that in neither case is this binding blocked by αIR-3, a highly specific monoclonal antibody to the type I receptor (48) (Figure 6). Under parallel conditions this antibody blocked approximately 70% of ^{125}I-Sm-C binding. These relationships were confirmed with highly purified preparations of the type I receptor, therefore suggesting that both Sm-C and IGF-II bind to the type I receptor, but at different binding sites that can be distinguished immunologically.

Table 2. Physical Characteristics and Hormonal Specificities of the Receptors for Insulin and the Somatomedin/Insulinlike Growth Factors

		Specificity for		
Receptor	Chemical structure	Insulin	Sm-C/IGF-I	IGF-II/MSA
Insulin	Unreduced: heterotetramer 300 KD Reduced subunits: α (binding): 130 KD β (tyrosine kinase): 90 KD	+ + + +	+	+ +
Type I (Sm-C/IGF-I)	Unreduced heterotetramer 300 KD Reduced subunits: α (binding): 130 KD β (tyrosine kinase): 90 KD	+	+ + + +	+ +
Type II (IGF-II/MSA)	Unreduced: 220 KD Reduced: 260 KD No known subunits	−[a]	+ +	+ + +

[a] Insulin stimulates increase in type II receptors on plasma membrane.
Source: Ref. 16.

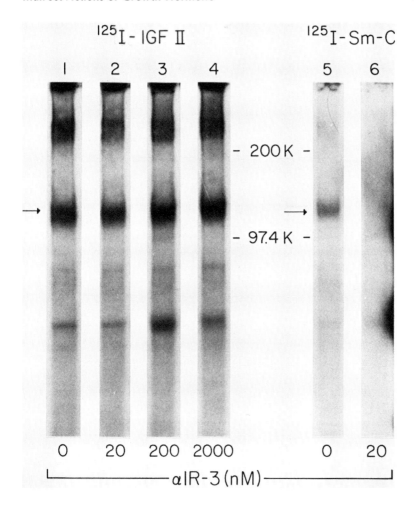

Figure 6. Effect of the anti–type I receptor antibody αIR-3 on binding of ^{125}I-IGF-II and ^{125}I-Sm-C/IGF-I to 130K binding site in human placental membranes. Particulate human placental membranes were incubated overnight at 4°C with ^{125}I-IGF-II (lanes 1–4) or ^{125}I-Sm-C (lanes 5 and 6) with graded concentrations of αIR-3 as shown on the figure, then affinity cross-linked with 0.3 mM disuccinimidyl suberate. Samples were solubilized, reduced, and analyzed by SDS-PAGE (3–14% gradient gel), then autoradiographed. The antibody blocked most of ^{125}I-Sm-C/IGF-I binding at a concentration of 20 nM, whereas concentrations up to 2000 nM failed to block binding of ^{125}I-IGF-II. (From Ref. 48.)

III. BIOLOGICAL ACTIONS OF SOMATOMEDINS

Effects of Somatomedins on Differentiation

The somatomedins often have as profound an effect on highly differentiated cell functions as they do on cell proliferation. Many of these
effects are primary responses to the growth factor and can be demonstrated in the absence of cell replication. In cartilage, somatomedin
stimulates synthesis of proteoglycans and other matrix elements (49);
in muscle it causes fusion of myoblasts into myotubes with a concomi-
tant increase in creatine kinase (26); in embryonic lens epithelium it
stimulates cell elongation and synthesis of delta crystallin (50); in
adipose tissue it stimulates lipoprotein lipase activity (51); and in granulosa cells it potentiates the action of FSH on the differentiation of
many cell-specific functions (52).

The effect of Sm-C on ovarian function was discovered by Dr.
Eli Adashi, who found that Sm-C greatly potentiated the actions of
FSH in rat granulosa cells on progesterone synthesis, induction of LH
receptors, and stimulation of aromatase activity (53) (Figure 7). Although the significance of these findings in the intact animal remains to
be clarified, the synergistic effect of Sm-C on FSH action could possibly explain why the administration of GH to some children with isolated GH deficiency appears to facilitate their pubertal development
(54).

Ewton and Florini showed in the L6 myoblast cell line that the
differentiation of myoblasts to myotubes is exquisitely sensitive to Sm-
C, but that at higher dosages this effect is reversed and thymidine
incorporation is stimulated (26).

In Vitro Growth-Promoting Actions of Somatomedin

Although somatomedins were first described as skeletal growth factors, they have been found to stimulate DNA synthesis and cell proliferation in a wide variety of cell types. These include fibroblasts,
sertoli, and granulosa cells, fetal liver cells, frog lens epithelium,
chondrocytes, smooth muscle and myoblasts, certain hematopoietic

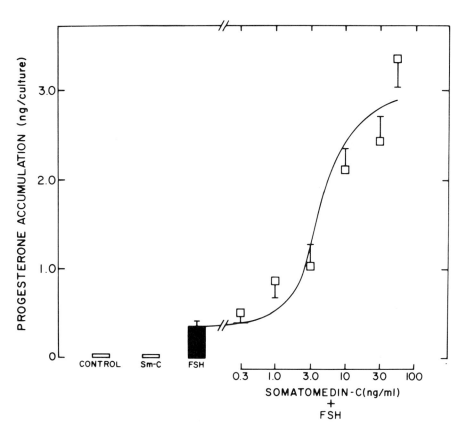

Figure 7. Synergism between Sm-C and FSH on progesterone accumulation by rat granulosa cells. Granulosa cells from immature hypophysectomized diethylstilbestrol-treated rats were cultured under serum-free conditions for 72 hours in the absence or presence of FSH (20 ng/ml), with or without increasing concentrations (0.1–50 ng/ml) of Sm-C. Collected media were assayed for their progesterone content by radioimmunoassay. The results represent the mean ±SEM of nine determinations representing triplicate measurements for each of three separate experiments. (From Ref. 53.)

lines, pituitary tumor cells, brain, and fetal limb buds. In many other types of cultured cells, the requirement for somatomedin can be satisfied by the inclusion of large amounts of insulin (55).

Somatomedin Is a Cell Cycle–Specific Mitogen

The effect of somatomedin on cell proliferation appears to be exercised primarily during the G_1 phase of the cell cycle. At confluency fibroblasts become arrested in G_0, but if they are then exposed to fresh serum derived from clotted blood they will enter G_1 and, after a minimal lag of 12 hours, reinitiate DNA synthesis. Platelet-poor plasma will not support traverse across G_1, however, since it lacks the platelet-derived growth factor (PDGF). If, however, quiescent Balb/c 3T3 cells are first exposed for a few hours to PDGF, they acquire the capability of responding to platelet-poor plasma and enter S phase after a lag of 12 hours (56). Plasma from GH-deficient donors is deficient in this mitogenic activity unless it is fortified with Sm-C (57) (Figure 8). With Pledger and Leof, we have shown that a combination of epidermal growth factor plus either nanomolar concentrations of somatomedin or micromolar concentrations of insulin is just as effective as platelet-poor plasma in stimulating PDGF-treated cells to traverse G_1 and enter DNA synthesis (58).

Immunoneutralization with Monoclonal Antibodies

The fact that a mixture of purified growth factors can mimic the action of plasma does not necessarily indicate that these are the physiologically important mitogens. A more elegant approach would be to selectively remove the putative growth factor from plasma with a monoclonal antibody. We have now accomplished this with highly specific monoclonal antibodies to Sm-C (designated sm 1.20) (59) and to the type I receptor (designated αIR-3) (60). As expected, sm 1.20 completely blocked the mitogenic effects of Sm-C + EGF but not the effect of EGF when high doses of insulin were used as a somatomedin surrogate (61). Of even greater significance was our finding that the antibody completely blocked the mitogenic effect of up to 10% platelet-poor plasma (Figure 9). This study left no doubt that Sm-C is an

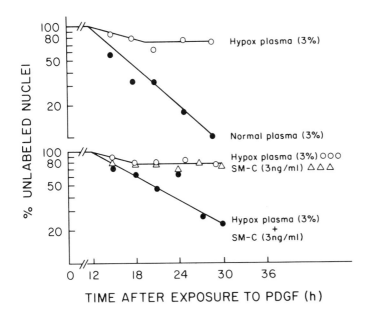

TIME AFTER EXPOSURE TO PDGF (h)

Figure 8. Studies demonstrating that the addition of pure Sm-C to hypophysectomized rat plasma restores progression factor activity. Quiescent, density-arrested cultures of Balb/c 3T3 cells were exposed for 3 hours to PDGF (25 ng/ml) in microtiter plates. After several washes, fresh medium containing 1 μCi of ^{3}H-thymidine was added to all cell cultures. At periodic intervals, DNA synthesis was arrested by the addition of 0.3 ml of 1 *M* ascorbic acid per milliliter of culture medium. The cells were subsequently fixed with methanol and processed for autoradiography. The data are plotted on a semilogarithmic scale as the fraction of unlabeled cell nuclei versus time after plasma addition. *Top*: The culture medium was supplemented with 3% plasma from either normal (closed circles) or hypophysectomized (open circles) rats. *Bottom*: Culture medium was supplemented with 3% plasma from hypophysectomized animals (open circles), 3% plasma from hypophysectomized animals plus 3 ng/ml of pure Sm-C (closed circles), or 3 ng/ml of pure Sm-C only (triangles). (From Ref. 57.)

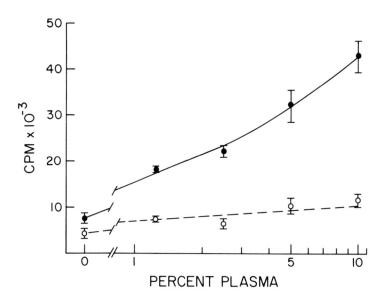

Figure 9. Quiescent Balb/c 3T3 fibroblasts were exposed to platelet-derived growth factor for 5 hours after which they were placed in the different concentrations of human platelet-poor plasma either in the presence (open circles) or absence (closed circles) of a 1:4000 dilution of monoclonal antibody to Sm-C. This study demonstrates that after selectively neutralizing Sm-C/IGF-I with a highly specific monoclonal antibody, human plasma is no longer mitogenic for Balb/c 3T3 cells. (From Ref. 61.)

essential constituent of the growth-promoting activity of human plasma and that after it is selectively removed, platelet-poor plasma is no longer mitogenic.

In further studies we were able to demonstrate that high concentrations of insulin induce mitogenesis in human fibroblasts by interacting with the type I receptor (62). In Figure 10 it is seen that the mitogenic effects of Sm-C on human fibroblasts are blocked both by antibody sm 1.20 directed toward Sm-C itself and by αIR-3, the antibody to the type I receptor, whereas the mitogenic effects of insulin are not blocked by sm 1.20 but are blocked by αIR-3.

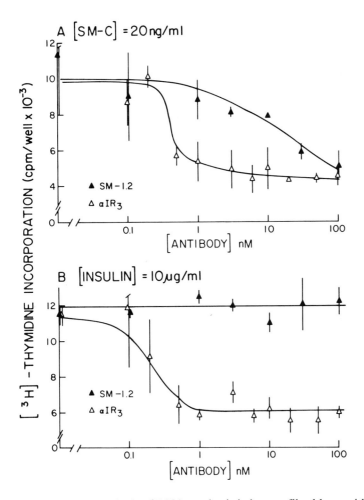

Figure 10. Blockade of DNA synthesis in human fibroblasts with αIR-3 and sm 1.2. Dose response of αIR-3 and sm 1.2 on Sm-C (top) or insulin (bottom) induced [³H]thymidine incorporation. (A) Confluent serum-starved human foreskin fibroblasts were exposed to background medium [Dulbecco's Modified Eagle's Medium; 0.5% (vol/vol) human hypopituitary plasma, and 100 nM dexamethansone] plus 20 ng/ml Sm-C and various doses of αIR-3 (open triangles) or sm 1.2 (closed triangles). (B) The same cells were exposed to background medium plus 10 μg/ml porcine insulin and various doses of αIR-3 (open triangles) or sm 1.2 (closed triangles). [³H]-thymidine was added 21 hours after the addition of hormone (with or without antibody). Acid-insoluble counts were harvested after 2 additional hours. The points are the mean ±SEM of values from triplicate wells in a representative experiment. Note that both antibodies blocked the mitogenic effect of Sm-C, whereas the mitogenic response to insulin was blocked only by the antireceptor antibody. (From Ref. 62.)

IV. ORIGIN OF SOMATOMEDINS IN MULTIPLE TISSUES

Evidence from Immunoneutralization Studies

An unanticipated byproduct of our studies with the monoclonal antibody to Sm-C was that it not only inhibited the mitogenic effects of the Sm-C + EGF combination in Balb/c 3T3 cells, but also partially inhibited the effect of EGF even when no Sm-C was added to the medium. Since the synergism between EGF and insulin in this system was not blocked, the antibody was clearly not blocking the effect of EGF itself, but rather was blocking the effects of small amounts of endogenously produced somatomedin. This was confirmed by finding that small amounts of somatomedinlike peptides were produced by Balb cells themselves (61). Subsequent studies revealed that the monoclonal antibody to Sm-C partially blocks the mitogenic effects of EGF and fibroblast growth factor in chicken heart mesenchymal cells (63), and the effect of PDGF in human fibroblasts and in porcine smooth muscle endothelial cells (64).

Evidence from Radioimmunoassay

These findings should have come as no surprise, since we are finding that given the appropriate circumstances, most any tissue can make somatomedinlike substances.

Production of Somatomedin by Fetal Tissues

Studies by D'Ercole et al. showed that a variety of fetal tissues produced somatomedinlike substances that are measurable in the radioimmunoassay for Sm-C. Media from organ explants obtained from 17-day mouse embryos revealed production of Sm-C–like substances by intestine, heart, brain, kidney, liver, and lung (65).

Production of Somatomedin by Tumors

Most of the established human tumor cell lines that we have successfully propagated in our laboratory in defined media have been found to make significant quantities of somatomedinlike substances,

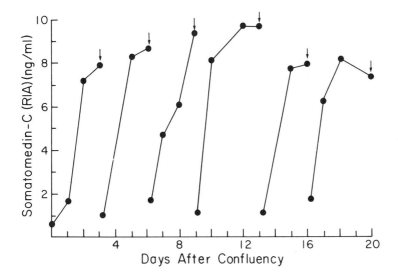

Figure 11. Production of somatomedin by cultures of a human mammary carcinosarcoma HS0578T. The tumor cell line was grown to confluency in 10-cm dishes, and the somatomedinlike immunoreactivity in the media was measured at the times shown by the Sm-C RIA. The conditioned media were harvested and replaced with new media every 3–4 days (arrows).

and we have identified several tumors that make substantially larger quantities than any normal cell line that we have studied (Figure 11). Bell and his co-workers found high levels of the mRNA for IGF-II in embryonic tissues and in Wilms' tumors of the kidneys (66,67).

Production by Human Fibroblasts

Human fibroblasts are seemingly not dependent on exogenous somatomedins for their growth since they are able to proliferate just as well in somatomedin-deficient serum as they are in serum from normal donors. Clemmons et al. found that human fibroblasts make their own somatomedin, and that this production is at least partly under growth hormone control (68,69).

V. CONTROL OF SOMATOMEDIN
PRODUCTION BY GROWTH HORMONE

Influence of Growth Hormone on Blood and Tissue Concentrations

Blood levels of Sm-C/IGF-I are markedly elevated in acromegaly and depressed in pituitary dwarfism, whereas blood levels of IGF-II are only moderately depressed in patients with GH deficiency and not elevated in acromegaly (70). Following the administration of GH to normal or hypopituitary subjects there is a delay of about 12 hours before there is any detectable rise in Sm-C/IGF-I blood levels, with peak values not being achieved until 20–30 hours after the GH administration (71).

Insight into the reason for this long delay in the induction of increased Sm-C/IGF-I blood levels was furnished by D'Ercole et al., who analyzed the somatomedin content in extracts from multiple tissues in normal and hypophysectomized rats, and the response of these levels to the administration of GH (72). After correcting the tissue extracts for the portion contributed by blood, the differences in Sm-C content between normal and hypox rats were striking except in the brain (Table 3). After GH administration the tissue levels of Sm-C rose many hours earlier than they did in blood, thus providing additional evidence that somatomedin in blood is derived from many different sources.

Growth Hormone Dependency of mRNAs for Sm-C and IGF-II in Rat Tissues

A more elegant demonstration of the GH dependency of the somatomedins has been made possible by the use of cDNA probes for human Sm-C and IGF-II provided for us by Drs. Leo Van den Brande and Maarten Jansen. With these probes we have been able to confirm that Sm-C is produced in many tissues in both the fetal and adult rat (73), and that, at least in the 100-g rat, the expression of the Sm-C gene is under strict GH control, whereas IGF-II is not except possibly in the brain (74).

Figure 12 shows Northern blots of Poly A+ RNA preparations of

Table 3. Extractable Tissue Sm-C Concentrations in Male Rats

| | Sm-C (U/g) | | |
| | Normal | Hypophysectomized | |
Tissue	Mean + SD	Mean + SD	% Normal
Serum	28.7 ± 0.98	0.74 ± 0.12	2.6
Liver	1.91 ± 0.23	0.23 ± 0.08	12.0
Lung	2.04 ± 0.86	0.57 ± 0.13	27.9
Kidney	2.59 ± 0.80	0.77 ± 0.29	29.7
Heart	0.92 ± 0.33	0.48 ± 0.14	52.2
Muscle (iliopsoas)	0.42 ± 0.05	<0.08	<19.1
Brain	0.26 ± 0.09	0.28 ± 0.04	107.7
Testes	1.88 ± 0.42	0.52 ± 0.32	27.7
Prostate	1.06	0.40	37.7
Thymus	0.33	0.10	30.3
Lymph nodes	0.48	0.08	16.7
Cartilage (sternum)	0.67	0.53	79.1
Fat pad (perirenal)	0.67 ± 0.19	0.25 ± 0.10	37.3
Submaxillary gland	1.73	0.78	45.1

Somatomedin-C/IGF-I content of tissues. Serum values are expressed as U/ml. Extractable immunoreactive Sm-C concentrations in tissues from normal and hypophysectomized rats. All values have been corrected for the contribution made by residual blood. All values, except for pooled organs, represent six or seven organs. Differences between Sm-C concentrations of normal and hypophysectomized rats are significant ($p < .005$). Values are pools of five or six organs.
Source: Ref. 72.

liver from three normal and hypophysectomized rats, and from three hypophysectomized rats 4 and 8 hours after the intraperitoneal administration of 200 μg of hGH. After electrophoresis and transfer to nitrocellulose paper, the separated RNAs were hybridized with probes for human Sm-C and IGF-II, with a ubiquitin cDNA (75) used as a control to ensure that the quantities of total poly A+ RNA were comparable in all specimens. In these animals the four Sm-C–specific messages were

Van Wyk et al.

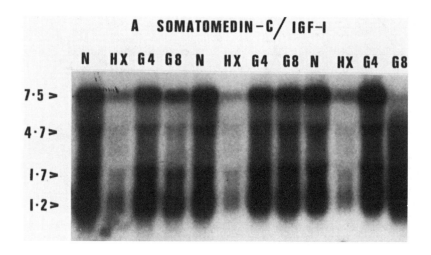

Figure 12. Growth hormone dependence of liver Sm-C/IGF-I mRNAs. Poly A+ RNAs were extracted from livers of three normal (N), hypophysectomized (HX), and hypophysectomized rats 4 hours (G4) or 8 hours (G8) after intraperitoneal injection of 200 μg (hGH). The poly A+ RNAs, each prepared from a different animal, were size fractionated on agarose gels, transferred to Gene Screen, and then hybridized with ^{32}P-labeled cDNA probes. Hybridization was at 42°C in a buffer containing 50% formamide, 5 × SSC, 5 × Denhardts, 0.5% SDS, 50 mM Tris-HCl pH 7.0, and 100 μg/ml salmon sperm DNA. After hybridization, blots were washed successively for 1 hour each in 2 × SSC, 0.5% SDS, 2 × SSC, and 0.1 × SSC at 65°C followed by exposure to x-ray film at −100°C with intensifying screens. (A) Blots were hybridized with a human Sm-C/IGF-I cDNA probe and exposed to x-ray film for 48 hours. (B) Replicate blot of the one shown in A was hybridized with a human IGF-II cDNA probe and exposed to x-ray film for 6 days. (C) To control for possible inequalities of mRNA from the respective animals the blot shown in A was stripped of hybridized Sm-C/IGF-I cDNA probe, rehybridized with a human ubiquitin cDNA probe (75) and exposed to x-ray film for 48 hours. Note that the small variations in the 3- and 3.5-kb ubiquitin mRNAs bear no discernible relationship to GH status. Numbers at the left of the blots are the estimated sizes of hybridizing mRNAs based on comparison with denatured Hind III fragments of lambda DNA electrophoresed on the same gels as the RNAs. (From Ref. 74.)

B IGF-II

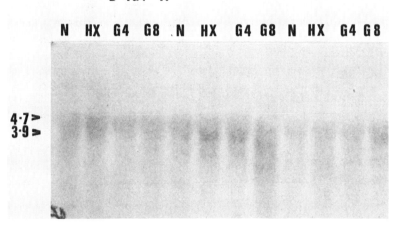

C UBIQUITIN

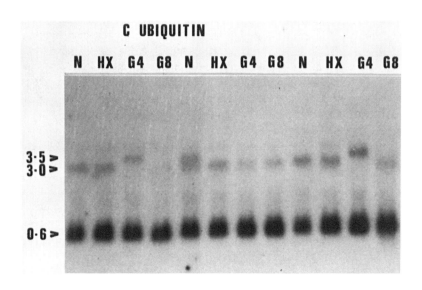

Figure 13.   Growth hormone dependence of Sm-C/IGF-I and IGF-II in rat pancreas and brain. Poly A+ RNAs were extracted from pancreas and brain of normal (N), hypophysectomized (HX), and hypophysectomized rats 4 hours (G4) or 8 hours (G8) after intraperitoneal injection of hGH as described in Figure 12. The poly A+ RNAs were size fractionated on agarose gels and transferred to Gene Screen. Hybridization and washing conditions were as described in Figure 12. Blots were exposed to x-ray film at −100°C with intensifying screens. Results are shown for only one representative animal, but similar results were obtained in the other similarly treated animals. *Top left*: Blots from pancreatic mRNA were hybridized with a human Sm-C/IGF-I cDNA probe and exposed to x-ray film for 6 days. The channel labeled B represents mRNA from a newborn rat pancreas, and the channel labeled WE represents mRNA from a whole 14-day rat embryo. *Top right*: Replicate blots of those above were hybridized with a human IGF-II cDNA probe and exposed to x-ray film for 6 days. *Bottom left*: To control for possible inequalities of mRNA from the respective animals, the blot of Sm-C/IGF-I mRNA shown above was stripped of hybridized Sm-C/IGF-I cDNA probe, rehybridized with cDNA probes for rat glucagon (1.3 kb), and somatostatin (0.7 kb) and exposed to x-ray film for 48 hours. *Bottom right*: Growth hormone dependence of brain IGF-II mRNAs. Blots were hybridized with a human IGF-II cDNA probe and exposed to x-ray film for 48 hours. There was no detectable mRNA for Sm-C/IGF-I in these preparations of rat brain. Comparisons with replicate blots that had been hybridized with a cDNA probe for ubiquitin suggested no cause other than GH dependency for the observed changes in abundance of brain IGF-II mRNA. Numbers at the left of the blots are the estimated sizes of hybridizing mRNAs based on comparison with denatured Hind III fragments of lambda DNA electrophoresed on the same gels as the RNAs. (From Ref. 74.)

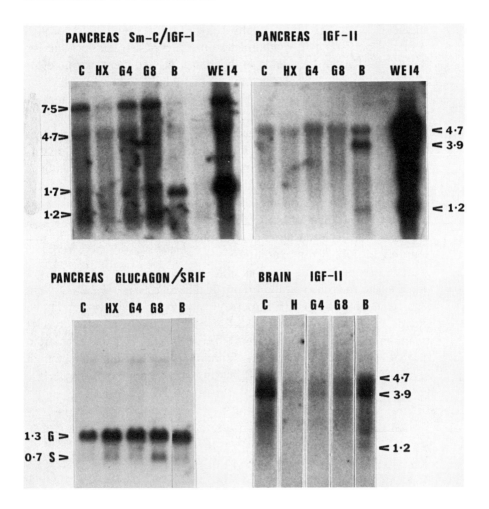

all greatly attenuated by hypophysectomy and restored essentially to normal 4 hours after GH administration. In contrast, the message for IGF-II was hardly discernible in the 100-g rat, and there was no clear change following hypophysectomy or GH administration.

The same four messages for Sm-C were seen in the pancreas of these animals (Figure 13), and, although the absolute levels were far lower than in the liver, they were similarly attenuated by hypophysectomy and restored 4 hours after GH administration. Also shown in this figure are Northern blots for Sm-C and IGF-II in the 14-day embryo and at birth. Very large quantities of message for both peptides were seen in the pancreas of 14-day embryos, with higher concentrations of those for IGF-II than for Sm-C/IGF-I, a relationship that is reversed in the 100-g rat. The glucagon control mRNAs were approximately the same in all poly A+ preparations.

A striking finding was that although in this study we could find no message for Sm-C in the brains of these 100-day rats, there were significant amounts of IGF-II message, and these levels appeared to be greatly attenuated by hypophysectomy and partially restored by GH treatment (Figure 13, bottom right). These data confirm and extend the data of Hasselbacher et al., who found that brain contained very high levels of immunoreactive IGF-II but little or no immunoreactive IGF-I (76).

VI. SUMMARY

It is becoming increasingly apparent that GH controls cellular differentiation and proliferation in many tissues through the local induction of Sm-C/IGF-I and to a lesser extent IGF-II. Nanomolar concentrations of these locally produced peptides act in concert with other growth factors to control growth by autocrine and paracrine mechanisms that are quite different from the humoral control mechanisms that classically trained endocrinologists have been accustomed to thinking about. Thus in designing future studies we must accommodate to the likelihood that in the living body the somatomedin that is produced proximal to the locus of its action will prove to be of greater biological importance than that arriving via the blood stream from a distal source.

REFERENCES

1. Salmon WD Jr, Daughaday WH. A hormonally controlled serum factor which stimulates sulfate incorporation by cartilage in vitro. J. Lab. Med. 49:825, 1957.

2. Daughaday WH, Reeder C. Synchronous activation of DNA synthesis in hypophysectomized rat cartilage by growth hormone. J. Lab. Clin. Med. 68:357–368, 1966.

3. Van Wyk JJ, Hall K, Van den Brande JL, Weaver RP. Further purification and characterization of sulfation factor and thymidine factor from acromegalic plasma. J. Clin. Endocrinol. Metab. 32:289, 1971.

4. Van Wyk JJ, Underwood LE, Hintz RL, Clemmons DR, Voina SJ, Weaver RP. The somatomedins: A family of insulin-like hormones under growth hormone control. Rec. Prog. Horm. Res. 30:259–318, 1974.

5. Rinderknecht E, Humbel RE. The amino acid sequence of human insulin-like growth factor I and its structural homology with proinsulin. J. Biol. Chem. 253:2769–2776, 1978.

6. Ellis S, Vodian MA, Grindeland RE. Studies on the bioassayable growth hormone-like activity of plasma. Rec. Prog. Horm. Res. 34:213–238, 1978.

7. Ashcraft MW, Hartzband PI, Van Herle AJ, Bersch N, Golde DW. A unique growth factor in patients with acromegaloidism. J. Clin. Endocrinol. Metab. 57:272–276, 1983.

8. Geffner ME, Bersch N, Kaplan SA, Lippe BM, Van Herle A, Elders MJ, Golde DW. Growth with growth hormone: Evidence for a potent circulating growth factor. Lancet 1:343–346, 1986.

9. Mittra I. Somatomedins and proteolytic bioactivation of prolactin and growth hormone. Cell 38:347–348, 1984.

10. Isaksson OGP, Eden S, Jansson J-O. Mode of action on pituitary growth hormone on target cells. Ann. Rev. Physiol. 47:483–499, 1985.

11. Golde DW. In vitro effects of growth hormone. In Growth Hormone and Other Biologically Active Peptides, Pecile A, Muller EE, eds., Excerpta Medica, Amsterdam, 1980, pp. 52–62.

12. Linzer DIH, Nathans D. Growth-related changes in specific mRNAs of cultured mouse cells. Proc. Natl. Acad. Sci. USA 80:4271–4275, 1983.

13. Linzer DIH, Lee S-J, Ogren L, Talamantes F, Nathans D. Identification of proliferation mRNA and protein in mouse placenta. Proc. Natl. Acad. Sci. USA 82:4356–4359, 1985.

14. Green H, Morikawa M, Nixon T. A dual effector theory of growth-hormone action. Differentiation 29:195–198, 1985.

15. Serrero G. Tumorigenicity associated with loss of differentiation and of response to insulin in the adipogenic cell line 1246. In Vitro Cell. Dev. Biol. 21:537–540, 1985.

16. Underwood LE, Van Wyk JJ. Normal and aberrant growth. In Williams Textbook of Endocrinology, 7th ed., Wilson JD, Foster DW, eds., Saunders, Philadelphia, 1985, pp. 155–205.

17. Fain JN, Kovacev VP, Scow RO. Effect of growth hormone and dexamethasone on lipolysis and metabolism in isolated fat cells of the rat. J. Biol. Chem. 240:3522, 1965.

18. Korner A. The induction of liver enzymes by growth hormone. In Growth and Growth Hormone, Pecile A, Muller E, eds., Excerpta Medica, Amsterdam, 1972, pp. 98–105.

19. Dawson CM, Hales CN. The effect of hypophysectomy on rat liver glucokinase activity and plasma glucose, insulin, and nonesterified fatty acid concentrations. Biochim. Biophys. Acta 184:287, 1969.

20. Richman RA, Underwood LE, Van Wyk JJ, Voina SJ. Synergistic effect of cortisol and growth hormone on hepatic ornithine decarboxylase activity. Proc. Soc. Exp. Biol. Med. 138:880, 1971.

21. Underwood LE, Van den Brande JL, Antony GJ, Voina SJ, Van Wyk JJ. Islet cell function and glucose homeostasis in hypopituitary dwarfism: Synergism between growth hormone and cortisone. J. Pediatr. 82:28–37, 1973.

22. Soyka LF, Crawford JD. Antagonism by cortisone of the linear growth induced in hypopituitary patients and hypophysectomized rats by human growth hormone. J. Clin. Endocrinol. Metab. 25:469, 1965.

23. Schoenle E, Zapf J, Humbel RE, Froesch ER. Insulin-like growth factor I stimulates growth in hypophysectomized rats. Nature 296:252–253, 1982.

24. Schoenle E, Zapf J, Froesch ER. Insulin-like growth factors I and II

stimulate growth of hypophysectomized rats. Diabetologia 23:199, 1982.

25. Brasel JA, Cheek DB. The effect of growth hormone on the cellular mass of hypopituitary dwarfs. In Growth Hormone, Pecile A, Muller E, eds., Excerpta Medica, Amsterdam, 1968, pp. 433–440.

26. Florini JR, Ewton DZ, Falen SL, Van Wyk JJ. Biphasic concentration dependency of stimulation of myoblast differentiation by somatomedins. Am. J. Physiol. (Cell Physiol. 19) 250:C1–C8, 1986.

27. Isaksson OGP, Jansson J-O, Gause IAM. Growth hormone stimulates longitudinal bone growth directly. Science 216:1237–1239, 1982.

28. Madsen K, Friberg U, Roos P, Isaksson O. Growth hormone stimulates the proliferation of cultured chondrocytes from rabbit ear and rib growth cartilage. Nature 304:545–547, 1983.

29. Abe H, Molitch M, Van Wyk JJ, Underwood LE. Human growth hormone and somatomedin-C suppress the spontaneous release of growth hormone in unanesthetized rats. Endocrinology 113:1319–1324, 1983.

30. Berelowitz M, Szabo M, Frohman LA, Firestone S, Chu L, Hintz RL. Somatomedin-C mediates growth hormone negative feedback by effects on both the hypothalamus and the pituitary. Science 212:1279–1281, 1981.

31. Brazeau P, Guillemin R, Ling N, Van Wyk JJ, Humbel R. Inhibion par les somatomedines de la secretion d l'hormone de croissance stimulee par le facteur hypothalamique somatocrinine (GRF) our le peptide de synthese hpGRF. C.R. Acad. Sci. 295(3):651–654, 1982.

32. Yamashita S, Melmed S. Insulin-like growth factor I action on rat anterior pituitary cells: Suppression of growth hormone secretion and messenger ribonucleic acid levels. Endocrinology 118:176, 1986.

33. Svoboda ME, Van Wyk JJ, Klapper DG, Fellows RE, Grissom FE, Schlueter RJ. Purification of Somatomedin-C from human plasma: Chemical and biological properties, partial sequence analysis, and relationship to other somatomedins. Biochemistry 19:790–797, 1980.

34. Klapper DG, Svoboda ME, Van Wyk JJ. Sequence analysis of somatomedin-C: Confirmation of identity with insulin-like growth factor I. Endocrinology 112:2215–2217, 1983.

35. Rinderknecht E, Humbel RE. Primary structure of human insulin-like growth factor II. FEBS Lett. 89:283–286, 1978.

36. Marquardt H, Todaro GJ, Henderson LE, Oroszlan S. Purification and primary structure of a polypeptide with multiplication-stimulating activity from rat liver cell cultures: Homology with human insulin-like growth factor II. J. Biol. Chem. 256:6859–6865, 1981.

37. Brissenden JE, Ullrich A, Francke U. Human chromosomal mapping of genes for insulin-like growth factors I and II and epidermal growth factor. Nature 310:781–784, 1984.

38. Dull TJ, Gray A, Hayflick JS, Ullrich A. Insulin-like growth factor II precursor gene organization in relation to insulin gene family. Nature 310:777–781, 1984.

39. Jansen M, van Schaik FMA, Ricker AT, Bullock B, Woods DE, Gabbay KH, Nussbaum AL, Sussenbach JS, Van den Brande JL. Sequence of cDNA encoding human insulin-like growth factor I precursor. Nature 306:609–611, 1983.

40. Rotwein P. Two insulin-like growth factor I messenger RNAs are expressed in human liver. Proc. Natl. Acad. Sci. USA 83:77–81, 1986.

41. Jansen M, van Schaik FMA, van Tol H, Van den Brande JL, Sussenbach JS. Nucleotide sequences of cDNAs encoding precursors of human insulin-like growth factor II (IGF-II) and an IGF-II variant. FEBS 179:243–246, 1985.

42. Hintz RL, Clemmons DR, Underwood LE, Van Wyk JJ. Competitive binding of somatomedin to the insulin receptors of adipocytes, chondrocytes, and liver membranes. Proc. Natl. Acad. Sci. USA 69:2351–2353, 1972.

43. Chernausek SD, Jacobs S, Van Wyk JJ. Structural similarities between human receptors for somatomedin-C and insulin: Analysis by affinity labeling. Biochemistry 20:7345–7350, 1981.

44. Massagué J, Czech MP. The subunit structures of two distinct receptors for insulin-like growth factors I and II and their relationship to the insulin receptor. J. Biol. Chem. 257:5036–5045, 1982.

45. Kasuga M, Van Obberghen E, Nissley SP, Rechler MM. Demonstration of two subtypes of insulin-like growth factor receptors by affinity cross-linking. J. Biol. Chem. 256:5405, 1981.

46. Oka Y, Mottola C, Oppenheimer CL, Czeck MP. Insulin activates the appearance of insulin-like growth factor II receptors on the adipocyte cell surface. Proc. Natl. Acad. Sci. USA 81:4028, 1984.

47. Mottola C, Czech MP. The type II insulin-like growth factor receptor does not mediate increased DNA synthesis in H-35 hepatoma cells. J. Biol. Chem. 259:12705, 1984.

48. Casella SJ, Han VK, D'Ercole AJ, Svoboda ME, Van Wyk JJ. Insulin-like growth factor binding to the type I somatomedin receptor: Evidence for two high affinity binding sites. J. Biol. Chem. 261:9268–9273, 1986.

49. Smeets T, Van Buul-Offers S. The influence of growth hormone, somatomedins, prolactin and thyroxine on the morphology of the proximal tibial epiphysis and growth plate on Snell dwarf mice. Growth 47:160, 1983.

50. Beebe DC, Silver M, Snellings KL, Van Wyk JJ. Structural and immunological similarities between lentropin, a factor that controls lens fiber differentiation, and insulin-like growth factors. Proc. Natl. Acad. Sci. USA 84:23–27, 1987.

51. Kern PA, Graves D, Baskin J, Eckel RH, Van Wyk JJ. Somatomedin-C may be a local regulator of lipoprotein lipase in human adipose tissue. Clin. Res. 33:62A, 1985.

52. Adashi EY, Resnick CE, D'Ercole AJ, Svoboda ME, Van Wyk JJ. Insulin-like growth factors as intraovarian regulators of granulosa cell growth and function. Endocrine Rev. 6:400–420, 1985.

53. Adashi EY, Resnick CE, Svoboda ME, Van Wyk JJ. A novel role for somatomedin-C in cytodifferentiation of the ovarian granulosa cell. Endocrinology 115:1227, 1984.

54. Laron Z, Mimouni F, Pertzelan A. Effect of human growth hormone therapy on penile and testicular size in boys with isolated growth hormone deficiency: First year of treatment. Isr. J. Med. Sci. 19:338, 1983.

55. Barnes D, Sato G. Methods for growth of cultured cells in serum-free medium. Anal. Biochem. 102:255, 1980.

56. Pledger WJ, Stiles CD, Scher CD, Antoniades HN. An ordered sequence of events is required before BALB/c 3T3 cells become committed to DNA synthesis. Proc. Natl. Acad. Sci. USA 75:2839, 1978.

57. Stiles CD, Capone GT, Scher CD, Antoniades HN, Van Wyk JJ, Pledger WJ. Dual control of cell growth by somatomedin and platelet derived growth factor. Proc. Natl. Acad. Sci. USA 76:1279–1284, 1979.

58. Leof EB, Wharton W, Van Wyk JJ, Pledger WJ. Epidermal growth factor and somatomedin-C regulate G_1 progression in competent BALB/c 3T3 cells. Exp. Cell. Biol. 141:107, 1982.

59. Gillespie GY, Van Wyk JJ, Underwood LE. Derivation of human monoclonal antibodies to human somatomedin-C/IGF-I. In Methods in Enzymology: Peptide Growth Factors, vol. 146, Barnes D, Sirbasku D, eds., Academic Press, Orlando, FL, 1987, pp. 207–216.

60. Kull FC Jr, Jacobs S, Su YU, Svoboda ME, Van Wyk JJ, Cuatrecasas P. Monoclonal antibodies to receptors for insulin and somatomedin-C. J. Biol. Chem. 258:6561–6566, 1983.

61. Russell WE, Van Wyk JJ, Pledger WJ. Inhibition of the mitogenic effects of plasma by a monoclonal antibody to somatomedin-C. Proc. Natl. Acad. Sci. USA 81:2389–2392, 1984.

62. Van Wyk JJ, Graves DC, Casella SJ, Jacobs S. Evidence from monoclonal antibody studies that insulin stimualtes deoxyribonucleic acid synthesis through the type I somatomedin receptor. J. Clin. Endocrinol. Metab. 61:639–643, 1985.

63. Balk SP, Morisi A, Gunther HS, Svoboda ME, Van Wyk JJ, Nissley SP, Scanes CG. Somatomedin (insulin-like growth factor) but not growth hormone are mitogenic for chicken heart mesenchymal cells and act synergistically with epidermal growth factor and brain fibroblast growth factor. Life Sciences 35:335–346, 1984.

64. Clemmons DR, Van Wyk JJ. Evidence for a functional role of endogenously produced somatomedin-like peptides in the stimulation of human fibroblast and porcine smooth muscle cell DNA synthesis. J. Clin. Invest. 75:1914–1918, 1985.

65. D'Ercole AJ, Applewhite GT, Underwood LE. Evidence that somatomedin is synthesized by multiple tissues in the fetus. Dev. Biol. 75:315, 1980.

66. Reeve AE, Eccles MR, Wilkins RJ, Bell GI, Millow LJ. Expression of insulin-like growth factor II transcripts in Wilms' tumour. Nature 317: 258–260, 1985.

67. Scott J, Cowell J, Robertson ME, Priestley LM, Wadey R, Hopkins B, Pritchard J, Bell GI, Rall LB, Knott TJ. Insulin-like growth factor-II gene expression in Wilms' tumour and embryonic tissues. Nature 317: 260–262, 1985.

68. Clemmons DR, Van Wyk JJ, Underwood LE. Hormonal control of somatomedin production by human fibroblasts. J. Clin. Invest. 67:10, 1981.

69. Clemmons DR, Van Wyk JJ. Somatomedin-C and platelet derived growth factor stimulate human fibroblast replication. J. Cell. Physiol. 106:361–367, 1981.

70. Clemmons DR, Van Wyk JJ. Factors controlling blood concentration of somatomedin-C. J. Clin. Endocrinol. Metab. 13:113–143, 1984.

71. Copeland KC, Underwood LE, Van Wyk JJ. Induction of immunoreactive somatomedin-C in human serum by growth hormone: Dose response relationships and effect on chromatographic profiles. J. Clin. Endocrinol. Metab. 50:690–697, 1980.

72. D'Ercole AJ, Stiles AD, Underwood LE. Tissue concentrations of somatomedin-C. Further evidence for multiple sites of synthesis and paracrine or autocrine mechanisms of action. Proc. Natl. Acad. Sci. USA 81:935–939, 1984.

73. Lund PK, Moats-Staats BM, Hynes MA, Simmons JG, Jansen M, D'Ercole AJ, Van Wyk JJ. Somatomedin-C/IGF-I and IGF-II mRNAs in rat fetal and adult tissues. J. Biol. Chem. 261:14539–14544, 1986.

74. Hynes MA, Van Wyk JJ, D'Ercole AJ, Jansen M, Lund PK. Growth hormone dependence of somatomedin-C/insulin-like growth factor I and insulin-like growth factor II messenger ribonucleic acids. Mol. Endocrinol. 1:233–242, 1987.

75. Lund PK, Moats-Staats BM, Simmons JG, Hoyt E, D'Ercole AJ, Van Wyk JJ. Nucleotide sequence analysis of a cDNA encoding human ubiquitin reveals that ubiquitin is synthesized as a precursor. J. Biol. Chem. 260:7609–7613, 1985.

76. Hasselbacher GK, Schwab ME, Pasi A, Humbel RE. Insulin-like growth factor II (IGF-II) in human brain: Regional distribution of IGF-II and of higher molecular mass forms. Proc. Natl. Acad. Sci. USA 82:2153–2157, 1985.

3

The Growth-Promoting Activity of Growth Hormone

JACK L. KOSTYO
University of Michigan Medical School
Ann Arbor, Michigan

Pituitary growth hormone (GH) is one of the principal hormones required for growth of the body during postnatal life, being absolutely essential for attainment of normal body size. The nature of the potent growth-promoting or anabolic action of GH has fascinated investigators for nearly six decades, and as a result, a sizable literature has accrued describing effects of the hormone on many aspects of the chemistry of the body. Indeed, many actions of the hormone have been described that are difficult to reconcile directly with its growth-promoting property. Besides stimulating the rate of somatic growth, GH can be diabetogenic when present in excess, causing hyperinsulinemia, insulin resistance, and increased glucose production by the liver. By contrast, in GH-deficient subjects or animals, GH exhibits transient insulinlike effects, stimulating glucose uptake and utilization by peripheral tissues, inhibiting hepatic glucose production, and inhibiting lipolysis in adipose tissue.

For many years, these diabetogenic and insulinlike effects of GH were attributed to contamination of the hormone with other pituitary substances having these biological properties. However, the recent availability of bacterially derived, biosynthetic GH, which is free of contamination with other pituitary substances, has made it possible to demonstrate that this is not the case. A number of laboratories have now shown that biosynthetic GH is both diabetogenic and insulinlike (for review, see refs. 1,2). These actions are therefore intrinsic biological properties of the hormone. Thus a fundamental question that must be addressed in any discussion of the biochemical means by which GH promotes growth is whether (and if so, how) the diabetogenic and insulinlike effects of GH are related mechanistically to its growth-promoting action.

I. DIABETOGENIC AND INSULINLIKE ACTIONS OF GH

A certain body of evidence, albeit indirect, suggests that the diabetogenic and insulinlike effects of GH are not related to its growth-promoting action. Research from several laboratories (for review, see refs. 3,4) on the structure–function relationships of human GH (hGH) have demonstrated that structural modification of the molecule can result in nonparallel shifts in the biological activity profile of the hormone, i.e., the ratios of growth-promoting:diabetogenic:insulinlike activities may vary depending on the structural change made in the molecule. For example, recent work (5) with the 20,000-dalton structural variant of GH (20-KD hGH) lacking amino acid residues 32–46 indicates that whereas the variant has full growth-promoting and diabetogenic activities, it has only 20% of the insulinlike activity of the 22,000-dalton form of the hormone. *S*-Carboxymethylated hGH has little growth-promoting or insulinlike activity, yet it retains high diabetogenic activity (6). Such nonparallel shifts in biological activity profile suggest that there are separate domains in the GH molecule for its several activities and hence structurally distinct receptors for each of these activities. Structural modifications in the molecule, such as those just referred to, presumably interfere in a differential manner with the various active site–receptor interactions. It should be pointed out, however, that to date there is no direct evidence for structural heterogeneity of GH receptors.

II. THE GH MOLECULE AND PROMOTION OF GROWTH

The active site for the growth-promoting property of GH resides in the N-terminal region of the molecule, proximal to amino acid 134. Studies (for review, see ref. 7) with large fragments of the N-terminal region of the hGH molecule have shown that these peptides have definite but weak growth-promoting activity. On the other hand, noncovalent complementation or recombination of hGH peptide 1-134 with various large peptides of the C-terminal third of the hGH molecule, which are themselves biologically inert, results in regeneration of substantial growth-promoting activity (for review, see refs. 8,9), indicating that a portion of the C-terminal of the molecule provides in some way for the expression of high growth-promoting activity. Precisely which region of the N-terminal of the GH molecule contains the domain for growth-promoting activity remains to be established. In any event, it does not embrace the region of the deletion in 20-KD hGH (residues 32–46), since the latter has full growth-promoting activity (10).

How does the interaction of this growth-promoting domain in the GH molecule with its receptor on target tissues lead to the stimulation of growth? To answer this question, it is necessary to define what is meant by *growth,* since GH exhibits such a multiplicity of biological effects, many'of which may or may not be related to its growth-promoting property. Arriving at a definition of growth as it pertains to the action of GH is difficult at best, and the dilemma involved was elegantly expressed by Paul Weiss in his introductory address for the Henry Ford Hospital International Symposium on ''The Hypophyseal Growth Hormone, Nature and Actions'' held in 1954. He said, ''Growth has come to connote any and all of these: reproduction, increase in dimensions, linear increase, gain in weight, gain in organic mass, cell multiplication, mitosis, cell migration, protein synthesis, and perhaps more'' (11). Certainly in the years preceding his statement and in the years that have followed, the growth-promoting action of GH has been described and quantitated in terms of many of these. For the present discussion, we define growth as cell multiplication, with the attendant protein and nucleic acid synthesis and cell division associated with that process.

Under this definition of growth, GH has been shown to exert growth-promoting effects on nearly every tissue of the body including cartilage, smooth and skeletal muscle, heart, liver, kidney, adipose tissue, lymphoid organs, and pancreatic β-cells among others, whereas the brain does not appear to be affected (for review, see ref. 12). Present knowledge of the cellular events associated with the stimulation by GH of growth in many of these target tissues has been derived mainly from experiments on hypophysectomized laboratory animals. It has been shown (for review, see refs. 12–14) that the administration of GH to such animals results in an array of effects on protein and nucleic acid metabolism, the earliest recognized events being enhanced transport of amino acids into the cells and a stimulation of the translation of pre-existing mRNA molecules for a variety of cellular proteins. These events are detectable within 30 minutes of the administration of GH (e.g., see ref. 15) and are transitory, lasting only 2–3 hours. Several hours after the administration of the hormone, the synthesis of various species of RNA, including ribosomal RNA, is stimulated, and, as a result, the protein synthetic capacity of the cell is greatly expanded. Eventually DNA synthesis is stimulated, and cell replication ensues.

III.   THE SOMATOMEDIN HYPOTHESIS OF GH ACTION

It has been difficult to duplicate this entire series of cellular events by the direct addition of GH to isolated tissues or organs. Indeed, only the rapid stimulatory effects of GH on amino acid transport and protein synthesis (translational) have been demonstrated routinely with the hormone in vitro, using certain tissues such as skeletal muscle, liver, heart, or fat. This and the observation that serum from GH-treated animals could stimulate the entire series of events in isolated cartilage gave rise to the generally held concept (16) that GH does not influence cell replication directly but does so indirectly by increasing the circulating concentration of potent mitogenic agents, the somatomedins, or insulinlike growth factors (in this case IGF-I), which are produced by the liver and other tissues in response to GH. Thus, according to this concept, the primary target organ for the growth-promoting action of GH would be the liver, and the other tissues of the body that grow in response to GH are not acted upon by the hormone directly.

To accept the somatomedin hypothesis, two issues must be reconciled. First, if GH only stimulates growth indirectly via IGF-I, what is the significance of the direct effects of GH on amino acid transport and protein synthesis that have been demonstrated in a number of tissues that do grow in response to GH? Are these effects produced in response to the growth-promoting action of GH, or are they a reflection of some other property of GH? Second, what is the physiological relevance of the specific binding sites for GH that have been demonstrated on the plasma membranes of many organs and tissues of the body, in addition to the liver? For example, when radioiodinated bovine GH or hGH is injected intravenously into the mouse, specific (i.e., displaceable) binding of the hormone can be demonstrated not only on membranes of liver, but also on membranes of heart, skeletal muscles, adipose tissue, lung, spleen, and pancreas (17; Kostyo, unpublished). Using isolated cells, specific binding sites for GH have been demonstrated not only on hepatocytes (for review, see ref. 18), but also on chondrocytes (19), adipocytes (20), rat insulinoma cells (21), various cultured preadipose cell lines (22), and cultured lymphocytes (23). What then is the function(s) of these binding sites for GH on nonhepatic cells? Do they actually play some role in mediating the growth-promoting action of GH, or are they involved only in the expression of the diabetogenic or insulinlike properties of the hormone? Two lines of recent work to be outlined provide some reconciliation of these issues with the somatomedin hypothesis and suggest that the latter may be an oversimplification of the mechanism by which GH stimulates growth.

IV. DIRECT EFFECTS OF GROWTH HORMONE

The first line of work deals with the question of whether the stimulatory effects of GH on amino acid transport and protein synthesis (translational), which occur within minutes after GH is administered or added directly to isolated tissues, are indeed expressions of the growth-promoting property of GH. In some respects, these actions of the hormone have characteristics similar to those of the insulinlike actions of GH on carbohydrate or lipid metabolism, e.g., they occur after a lag phase of 20–30 minutes, they last only 2–3 hours, and they are readily demonstrable only in GH-deficient animals. Thus they might in fact be expressions of the insulinlike property of GH and be mediated by the putative receptors for this action of the hormone. The recent finding (5) that 20-KD hGH has only 20% the insulinlike activity of 22-KD hGH, while retaining full growth-promoting and diabetogenic activities, suggested that it would be an excellent reagent to test the preceding hypothesis.

If the rapid, direct effects of GH on amino acid transport and protein synthesis are reflections of the growth-promoting property of GH, then one might expect 20-KD hGH to be as active as 22-KD hGH in eliciting these effects. On the other hand, if they are reflections of the insulinlike action of GH, 20-KD hGH should be much less active in stimulating amino acid transport and protein synthesis than 22-KD hGH. To test the hypothesis, we (Kostyo et al., unpublished) used the isolated, intact hemidiaphragm preparation of the hypophysectomized rat, which responds reproducibly to GH added in vitro not only with enhanced amino acid transport and protein synthesis but also with enhanced sugar transport, reflecting the insulinlike action of GH. The isolated diaphragms were incubated in the absence or presence of various concentrations of either native 22-KD hGH or a highly purified native 20-KD hGH preparation, and the effects of these hormones on 3-*O*-methylglucose transport, α-aminoisobutyric acid transport, and phenylalanine incorporation into protein were measured. As expected, the 20-KD hGH preparation was approximtely 20% as effective as 22-KD hGH in stimulating 3-*O*-methylglucose transport into the diaphragm, reflecting its markedly attenuated insulinlike activity. Similarly, the 20-KD hGH preparation was only 20% as effective as 22-KD hGH in stimulating α-aminoisobutyric acid transport and phenylalanine incorporation into protein in the same muscles. This evidence favors the conclusion that the rapid stimulatory actions of GH on amino acid transport and the translation of preexisting mRNA are expressions of the insulinlike action of the hormone, presumably mediated via a population of receptors for this property of GH. These effects, therefore, are probably not components of the response of target cells to the growth-promoting action of GH.

The second line of recent work bears on the question of whether GH itself has any direct growth-promoting action, or whether its effect on growth is mediated by circulating insulinlike growth factors. It is well established that GH deficiency causes a marked decrease in the rate of longitudinal bone growth and that the administration of GH to

GH-deficient animals restores the rate of bone growth to normal. The action of GH on longitudinal bone growth is to stimulate the proliferation of chondrocytes in the epiphyseal growth plate. Early attempts to show in vitro effects of GH on DNA synthesis or other aspects of cartilage metabolism were unsuccessful, whereas plasma obtained from GH-treated hypophysectomized animals did have in vitro stimulatory effects on cartilage metabolism. It was subsequently demonstrated that the stimulatory factors in plasma responsible for these effects were the somatomedins or insulinlike growth factors (for review, see ref. 16). These findings established the somatomedin hypothesis of GH action, which proposed that GH stimulates cell replication and growth indirectly by stimulating the production of IGFs.

A number of recent observations challenge the idea that it is the rise in circulating IGFs that mediates GH's action on chrondrocyte proliferation. For example, it has been shown (24–26) that the injection or infusion of GH directly into the epiphyseal growth plate of one of the tibia of the hypophysectomized rat stimulates longitudinal growth of the bone. The contralateral tibia, which is not injected, does not grow when low concentrations of GH are employed. Thus it has been concluded that GH can exert a local effect on bone growth, presumably by acting on chondrocytes directly. Additional observations support this conclusion. It has been shown (19,27) that chondrocytes isolated from rabbit epiphyseal, ear, and articular cartilage possess specific binding sites for GH. It has also been shown (28) that GH added in vitro can stimulate DNA synthesis in cultured rat and rabbit chondrocytes, an event that requires a number of hours to become manifest. Further, Lindahl et al. (29) recently showed that hGH added to cultures of rat tibial chondrocytes suspended in agarose stimulates the formation of large colonies of these cells within 10–14 days after addition of the hormone to the culture medium. These authors propose that GH acts preferentially on stem cell chondrocytes or early proliferative chondrocytes that have a high capacity to proliferate, and that the subsequent clonal growth of these cells may be dependent upon the autocrine or paracrine action of IGFs produced by the chondrocytes themselves.

The conclusion that GH may act on only certain chondrocytes in the cartilage growth plate is supported by recent studies by Isaksson et al. (12), who examined the specific binding of radioiodinated hGH to chondrocytes in rat rib growth plates in vitro. Autoradiography revealed that the hGH was bound to chondrocytes only in the germinal zone, and none was bound to chondrocytes in the proliferative or hypertrophic zones of the growth plate. They conclude that GH acts primarily on the prechondrocytes in the germinal zone. Further, they proposed that the action of GH on these cells is to stimulate them to differentiate into chondrocytes, which then undergo the proliferation that leads to longitudinal bone growth.

One of the differentiative events is presumed (12) to be the expression of genes coding for IGF-I. This factor would then act either in an autocrine or paracrine manner on the differentiated chondrocyte to stimulate it to undergo clonal expansion. Preliminary evidence from Isaksson's laboratory (30) supports this conclusion. Using immunofluorescence to localize IGF-I, these investigators found that chondrocytes in the proliferative zone of the rat epiphyseal growth plate fluoresced brightly, whereas those in the germinal and hypertropic zones did not. Hypophysectomy greatly reduced the number of cells in the proliferative area that contained immunoreactive material, and GH administration restored the number of fluorescing cells toward normal, suggesting that it stimulates the synthesis of IGF-I in these cells. Whether this is indeed the case remains to be established.

V. SUMMARY

The foregoing evidence suggests that GH exerts its growth-promoting action on longitudinal bone growth directly, by stimulating the differentiation of prechondrocytes into cells that can produce IGFs and then respond to the mitogenic actions of these substances (12). Indeed, this concept of the growth-promoting action of GH probably applies generally to its actions on the growth of many tissues of the body, as Green and his colleagues eloquently stated (31). Many cells of the body are probably direct targets for the growth-promoting action of GH, and the basis for this action is to cause the cells to differentiate into a form capable of responding to the mitogenic action of other growth factors and/or to induce within the cells the capability to produce growth factors to which they can then respond. Future work will be required to establish whether this altered view of the growth-promoting action of GH is indeed correct and to define the molecular events that are involved.

REFERENCES

1. Kostyo JL, Gennick SE, Sauder SE. Diabetogenic activity of native and biosynthetic human growth hormone in obese (ob/ob) mouse. Am. J. Physiol. 246:E356–E360, 1984.

2. Goodman HM, Grichting G, Coiro V. Growth hormone action on adipocytes. In Human Growth Hormone, Raiti S, Tolman RA, eds., Plenum, New York, 1986, pp. 499–512.

3. Goodman HM, Kostyo JL. Altered profiles of biological activity of growth hormone fragments on adipocyte metabolism. Endocrinology 108:553–558, 1981.

4. Gennick SE, Kostyo JL, Mills JB, Edén S. A hybrid noncovalent complex of fragments of porcine and human growth hormones with diabetogenic activity. Endocrinology 112:2069–2075, 1983.

5. Kostyo JL, Cameron CM, Olson KC, Jones AJS, Pai R-C. Biosynthetic 20-kilodalton methionyl-human growth hormone has diabetogenic and insulin-like activities. Proc. Natl. Acad. Sci. USA 82:4250–4253, 1985.

6. Cameron CM, Kostyo JL, Rillema JA, Gennick SE. Reduced and S-carboxymethylated human growth hormone: A probe for diabetogenic action. Am. J. Physiol. 247:E639–644, 1984.

7. Mills JB, Kostyo JL, Reagan CR, Wagner SA, Moseley MH, Wilhelmi AE. Fragments of human growth hormone produced by digestion with thrombin: Chemistry and biological properties. Endocrinology 107:391–399, 1980.

8. Reagan CR, Kostyo JL, Mills JB, Gennick SE, Messina JL, Wagner SA, Wilhelmi AE. Recombination of fragments of human growth hormone: Altered activity profile of the recombinant molecule. Endocrinology 109:1663–1671, 1981.

9. Thorson JA, Sauder SE, Gennick SE, Kostyo JL, Mills JB. Complementation of human growth hormone (GH) peptide 1-134 with C-terminal fragments of human GH produced by digestion with bromelain. Endocrinology 112:782–787, 1983.

10. Lewis UJ, Dunn JT, Bonewald LF, Seavey BK, VanderLaan WP. A naturally occurring structural variant of human growth hormone. J. Biol. Chem. 253:2679–2687, 1978.

11. Weiss P. What is growth? In The Hypophyseal Growth Hormone, Nature and Actions. Smith RW Jr, Gaebler OH, Long CNH, eds., McGraw-Hill, New York, 1955, pp. 3–16.

12. Isaksson OGP, Edén S, Jansson J-O. Mode of action of pituitary growth hormone on target cells. Ann. Rev. Physiol. 47:483–499, 1985.

13. Kostyo JL, Nutting DF. Growth hormone and protein metabolism. In Handbook of Physiology, Section 7: Endocrinology IV, Part 2, Williams and Wilkins, Baltimore, 1974, pp. 187–210.

14. Kostyo JL, Isaksson O. Growth hormone and the regulation of somatic growth. In International Review of Physiology, Reproductive Physiology II, Vol. 13, University Park Press, Baltimore, 1977, pp. 255–274.

15. Dreskin SC, Kostyo JL. Acute effects of growth hormone on the function of ribosomes of rat skeletal muscle. Horm. Metab. Res. 12:60–66, 1980.

16. Daughaday WD. Growth hormone and the somatomedins. In Endocrine Control of Growth, Daughaday WD, ed., Elsevier, New York, 1981, pp. 1–24.

17. Ciccia-Torres GN, Turyn D, Dellacha JD. Mouse liver specific uptake of iodinated growth hormones: Evidence for the presence of somatogenic and lactogenic sites. Horm. Metab. Res. 15:443–448, 1983.

18. Messina JL, Edén S, Kostyo JL. Effects of hypophysectomy and GH administration on bovine and human GH binding to rat liver membranes. Am. J. Physiol. 249:E56–E62, 1985.

19. Edén S, Isaksson OGP, Madsen K, Friberg U. Specific binding of growth hormone to isolated chondrocytes from rabbit ear and epiphyseal plate. Endocrinology 112:1127–1129, 1983.

20. Fagin KD, Lackey SL, Reagen CR, DiGirolamo M. Specific binding of growth hormone by rat adipocytes. Endocrinology 107:608–615, 1980.

21. Billestrup N, Martin JM. Growth hormone binding to specific receptors stimulates growth and function of cloned insulin-producing rat insulinoma RIN-5AH cells. Endocrinology 116:1175–1181, 1985.

22. Nixon T, Green H. Properties of growth hormone receptors in relation to the adipose conversion of 3T3 cells. J. Cell. Physiol. 115:291–295, 1983.

23. Lesniak MA, Gorden P, Roth J, Gavin JR III. Binding of ^{125}I-human growth hormone to specific receptors in human cultured lymphocytes. J. Biol. Chem. 249:1661–1667, 1974.

24. Isaksson OGP, Jansson J-O, Gause IAM. Growth hormone stimulates longitudinal bone growth directly. Science 216:1237–1239, 1982.

25. Russell S, Spencer M. Local injections of human or rat growth hormone or of purified somatomedin-C stimulate unilateral tibial epiphyseal growth in hypophysectomized rats. Endocrinology 116:2563–2567, 1985.

26. Isgaard J, Nilsson A, Lindahl A, Jansson J-O, Isaksson OGP. Effects of local administration of GH and IGF-I on longitudinal bone growth in rats. Am. J. Physiol. 250:E367–E372, 1986.

27. Postel-Vinay MD, Corvol MT, Lang F, Fraud F, Guyda H, Posner B. Receptors for insulin-like growth factors in rabbit articular and growth plate chondrocytes in culture. Exp. Cell. Res. 148:105–116, 1983.

28. Madsen K, Friberg U, Roos P, Edén S, Isaksson O. Growth hormone stimulates the proliferation of cultured chondrocytes from rabbit ear and rat rib growth cartilage. Nature 304:545–547, 1983.

29. Lindahl A, Isgaard J, Nilsson A, Isaksson OGP. Growth hormone potentiates colony formation of epiphyseal chondrocytes in suspension culture. Endocrinology 118:1843–1848, 1986.

30. Nilsson A, Isgaard J, Lindahl A, Dahlström A, Isaksson OGP. Growth hormone increases the number of chondrocytes containing IGF-I/Sm-C immunoreactive material in the rat epiphyseal growth plate. Acta Physiol. Scand. 124 (Suppl 542):323, 1985. (abstract)

31. Green H, Morikawa M, Nixon T. A dual effector theory of growth-hormone action. Differentiation 29:195–198, 1985.

4

Biochemical Basis for the Lipolytic Activity of Growth Hormone

H. MAURICE GOODMAN, ERELA GORIN,*
and THOMAS W. HONEYMAN
University of Massachusetts Medical School
Worcester, Massachusetts

A relationship between growth hormone (GH) and the metabolism of lipids has been suspected since the early 1930s when Lee and Shaeffer (1) demonstrated that prolonged treatment of rats with pituitary extracts that were rich in growth-promoting activity produced a relative decrease in total carcass fat while promoting an overall increase in body size. Various other studies led to the proposals that the pituitary gland contained a ketogenic principle, a fat-metabolizing factor, and a

*Current affiliation: Faculty of Medicine, Technion, Haifa, Israel.

These studies were supported by grant AM 19392 from the National Institutes of Health.

specific metabolic principle (2–6). Investigations with grossly impure preparations clearly demonstrated that some pituitary principle or principles, when administered in what we now know to be very large doses, increased the accumulation of fat in the liver and produced gross lipemia (2–6). Experiments with deuterium-labeled fat left little doubt that the lipids that accumulated in the liver arose in adipose tissue (7,8). With the isolation of purified GH (9,10), it became apparent that GH itself was the principle responsible for the loss of carcass fat (11–16) and the various "adipokinetic" activities present in crude pituitary extracts.

Progress in understanding the role of GH in fat mobilization awaited the recognition that free fatty acids (FFA) are the physiological form in which fat is mobilized from adipose tissue (17,18). Raben and Hollenberg (19) were the first to demonstrate that GH increased the concentration of FFA in the plasma of fasting dogs and human subjects. Their findings have been confirmed in a wide variety of mammalian species (see ref. 3 for review). In general, it has been observed that the increase in plasma FFA after a single injection of GH requires a lag period of 2 or more hours. While consistent responses have been seen in many species, the amount of GH needed to produce measurable increases in plasma levels of FFA has been quite high: GH doses of 5–10 mg/kg have usually been used to demonstrate increased mobilization of FFA in rats (20–24), and although lower doses have been found effective in fasting human subjects (19,25–27) and rhesus monkeys (28), the doses used (0.014–3.0 mg/kg) nevertheless still exceed what can be reasonably considered physiological. More recently, however, Gerich et al. (29) found that in properly prepared patients, a sustained infusion of GH at a rate that maintained plasma levels of GH within the normal range at about 6 ng/ml more than doubled plasma concentrations of FFA and glycerol. In these studies, the concentrations of glucagon, insulin, or GH were held constant by suppressing endogenous secretion with somatostatin, while simultaneously infusing these hormones at constant rates. These studies revealed not only that physiologically relevant amounts of GH can increase lipolysis in vivo, but also that compensatory increases or decreases in the secretory rates of other hormones, which have overlapping or antagonistic effects, can mask the effects of GH.

Attempts to demonstrate lipolytic effects of GH in vitro using segments of epididymal fat from the rat or isolated adipocytes produced disappointing results and raised doubts as to whether GH actually was lipolytic. While hormones such as epinephrine, ACTH, and TSH produced fivefold to 10-fold increases in lipolysis virtually instantaneously (30), even very high concentrations of GH appeared to have little effect. It was only with the recognition that the lipolytic effects of GH are slow in onset and require the presence of other agents such as glucocorticoids (31) or theophylline (32) that convincing lipolytic effects were demonstrable with any degree of consistency. Nevertheless, variability in the responses seen with different preparations of GH, tissues of different animal species, and experimental conditions from lab to lab nurtured lingering doubts about whether it was GH itself or trace contaminants that produced delayed lipolytic activity. These doubts were finally set to rest with the demonstration that hGH produced in bacteria through recombinant DNA technology and hence free of contamination with any pituitary peptides has indisputable intrinsic lipolytic potency (33,34).

I. THE PROCESS OF LIPOLYSIS

Before exploring the lipolytic actions of GH, it will be useful to review current understanding of the lipolytic process as summarized in Figure 1 (see refs. 35 and 36 for review). Lipids are stored in adipose tissue in the form of triglycerides which are comprised of 3 mol of long-chain fatty acids in ester linkage with 1 mol of glycerol. Lipolysis is the stepwise enzymatic cleavage of the ester bonds to release fatty acids and glycerol. The rate-determining step appears to be the cleavage of the ester bond at the α-carbon of glycerol and is catalyzed by the hormone-sensitive lipase. Successive cleavage by the hormone-sensitive lipase or other tissue esterases progresses rapidly, with little or no accumulation of mono- and diglycerides. Only a small fraction of the fatty acids released from ester linkage escape from the adipocyte to become the FFA of the blood. The majority, usually more than two-thirds, are reesterified and hence trapped in the fat cell as triglyceride. The net rate of FFA mobilization is determined by the relative rates of the opposing processes of lipolysis and reesterification. Although the fatty acids released by lipolysis can be recycled into triglycerides, the glycerol cannot be reutilized and escapes into the extracellular space. Therefore, the rate of production of glycerol (rather than fatty acids) provides a good index of lipolysis, and will be so used in the studies presented here.

The reesterification reaction requires that the glycerol be in the

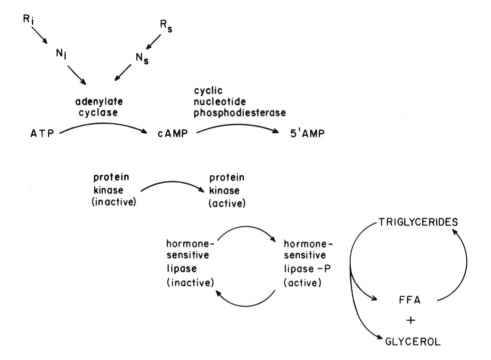

Figure 1.   Biochemical reactions in lipolysis in adipose tissue.

form of α-glycerol phosphate. Free glycerol produced by lipolysis cannot be phosphorylated and used for reesterification because adipocytes are deficient in the enzyme α-glycerokinase (37). The only source of α-glycerol phosphate is the triose phosphate pool which is derived from glucose metabolism. The rate of fatty acid release thus is sensitive to any factor that affects the rate of glucose metabolism in adipocytes. In addition to promoting lipolysis, as discussed later, GH increases the fraction of fatty acids that escape from the cells as FFA (38) because it limits the availability of α-glycerol phosphate for reesterification by decreasing glucose metabolism in adipocytes (39). Inhibition of reesterification can theoretically double or triple the rate of FFA mobilization even if the rate of lipolysis is unchanged.

The hormone-sensitive lipase, which is an 84,000-dalton protein, appears to be regulated by the reversible phosphorylation of a single serine residue (40). Phosphorylation, which activates the enzyme, is catalyzed by the cyclic AMP–dependent protein kinase (protein kinase A). Even in the absence of hormonal stimulation, this enzyme, or perhaps an additional triglyceride lipase, appears always to be at least partially active, for the rate of glycerol release from adipocytes rarely falls to zero. Similarly, adenylate cyclase, the enzyme that catalyzes the formation of cAMP from ATP, also appears always to be at least partially activated. Adenylate cyclase is the catalytic component of a variety of hormone receptor complexes in the adipocyte membrane. These hormone receptor complexes consist of at least two additional components: the recognition subunits, which bind stimulatory or inhibitory agonists, and the guanine nucleotide binding subunits, which couple the catalytic component to recognition components. The guanine nucleotide binding proteins, called G proteins by some authors and N proteins by others, apparently play a regulatory role in many cell types (41–43).

II. THE ROLE OF HORMONES IN THE REGULATION OF LIPOLYSIS

The adipocyte, which is endocrinologically promiscuous, can respond to a wide range of endocrine and paracrine signals that may be either stimulatory or inhibitory. Stimulatory agonists such as epinephrine bind to the stimulatory recognition unit, designated R_s in Figure 1. When an agonist binds to R_s, the coupled nucleotide binding subunit, designated N_s, is induced to bind a molecule of GTP in exchange for a molecule of GDP (41–43). This has the dual effect of decreasing the affinity of R_s for the agonist and increasing the activity of adenylate cyclase. R_s also catalyzes the conversion of GTP to GDP, and in so doing restores the resting state. Essentially the same sequence of events occurs when the inhibitory recognition subunits, R_i, bind to such inhibitory agonists as adenosine or the prostaglandins. In this case, upon binding GTP, the nucleotide-binding coupling protein, N_i, exerts an inhibitory action on adenylate cyclase (41–43).

The activity of adenylate cyclase expressed at any moment therefore is determined by the balance struck between stimulatory and inhibitory agonists (Figure 2). The relatively inactive state of the enzyme seen under resting "basal" conditions in human and rat adipose tissue appears to result from the predominance of inhibitory influences which dampen the behavior of an intrinsically active molecule, rather than

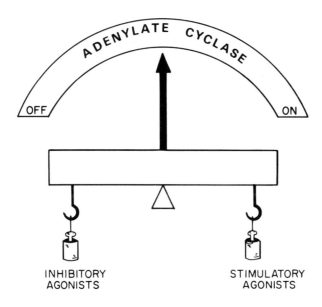

Figure 2. Interaction of stimulatory and inhibitory factors in the regulation of adenylate cyclase activity.

from the lack of stimulation of an intrinsically inactive molecule. Production of prostaglandins from endogenous arachidonate (44,45) and adenosine (46–50) from adenine nucleotides appears to be ongoing. The latter is more readily demonstrable in isolated adipocytes than in tissue segments (50). Even in the absence of stimulatory input, inhibition of prostaglandin formation, hastening of adenosine destruction, or blockade of the N_i which mediates their effects results in a progressive increase in lipolysis, reflective of adenylate cyclase activity (46).

Interaction with R_s or R_i to stimulate or inhibit the activity of adenylate cyclase is not the only way that hormones can affect lipolysis. An enzyme, cyclic nucleotide phosphodiesterase, which catalyzes the degradation of cAMP, is activated by insulin (51). The activity of this enzyme is also increased in tissues of adrenalectomized (52) or thyroidectomized (53) animals and restored by treatment with glucocorticoids or thyroxine, suggesting that its turnover may be regulated by these hormones. Some evidence suggests that insulin may limit lipolysis at a site or in a manner that is independent of cAMP concentrations (36). Other evidence suggests that thyroid hormones may affect the synthesis or turnover of the stimulatory receptor in some tissues (54), and it is possible that turnover of the hormone-sensitive lipase itself may be subject to hormonal regulation.

III. GROWTH HORMONE AND LIPOLYSIS

The precise way in which GH affects lipolysis has not yet been defined. As already indicated, the lipolytic effects of GH are slow to develop and are most readily demonstrated under circumstances that favor lipid mobilization, such as fasting (3) or, in vitro, in the presence of another agent, such as a glucocorticoid (Figure 3). The data shown were obtained by incubating segments of rat epididymal fat in standard incubation medium in the presence of glucose, bovine serum albumin, and GH, dexamethasone, or both. The tissues were transferred to fresh incubation medium every hour, and the glycerol content was measured to determine the rate of lipolysis each hour. The rate of glycerol production during the first hour was unaffected by any of the hormones and was relatively brisk. In the second, third, and fourth hours, the basal rate of glycerol release was diminished, and it was unaffected by either GH alone or dexamethasone alone. The combination of the two hormones, however, produced a highly significant increase in glycerol production that became evident in the second hour and was pronounced in the fourth hour.

To determine the dose dependency of the response, tissues were preincubated for 3 hours in the presence of 100 ng/ml of dexamethasone and various concentrations of bovine GH ranging from 1 to 100 ng/ml (Figure 4). Glycerol production was measured in the fourth hour of incubation. A statistically significant effect of GH was seen with as little as 1 ng/ml, with a maximum response observed at about 30–100 ng/ml. The GH preparation used for these experiments was the international standard for bovine GH and, by definition, contained 1 U/ml. The data shown were obtained as part of an international collaborative study to establish a standard for human GH. The GH preparations used in some of the other studies have about 2 international units of activity per milligram. These data indicate that concentrations of GH corre-

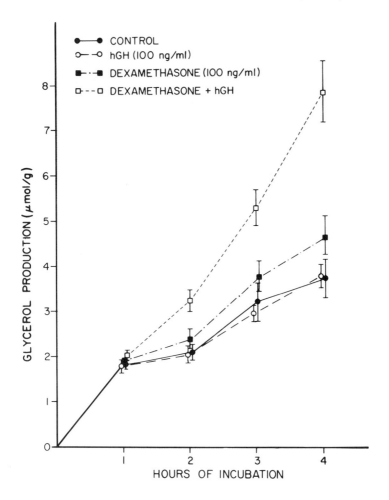

Figure 3.   Effects of GH and dexamethasone on lipolysis. Segments of epididymal adipose tissue obtained from eight normal rats were incubated in Krebs Ringer bicarbonate buffer containing 4% bovine serum albumin and 5.5 mM glucose along with hGH or dexamethasone. At the end of each hour for 3 hours, the tissues were transferred to fresh incubation medium of identical composition and reincubated for an additional hour. Glycerol produced in each hour was measured enzymatically and added to that produced in the previous hour to give the cumulative output over the entire 4 hours. Each point is the mean of eight observations. The standard errors are indicated by the vertical brackets. The effects of GH and dexamethasone were statistically significant ($p < .05$) after 2 hours.

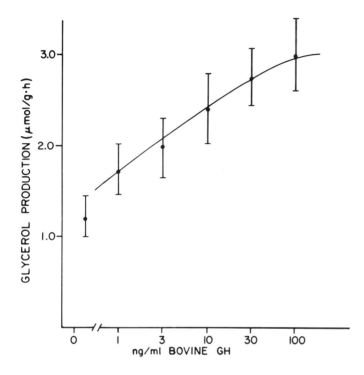

Figure 4. Dose–response relationship for the lipolytic effects of GH in the presence of dexamethasone. Segments of adipose tissues from normal rats were preincubated for 3 hours in the presence of 100 ng/ml of dexamethasone and concentrations of bovine GH that ranged from 0 to 100 ng/ml. The tissues were then transferred to fresh medium for measurement of glycerol production in the fourth hour. Each point represents the mean of 16 observations. The vertical brackets indicate the standard errors. Statistically significant effects ($p < .05$) were produced by 1 ng/ml or higher concentrations as judged by Duncan's multiple range test after analysis of variance.

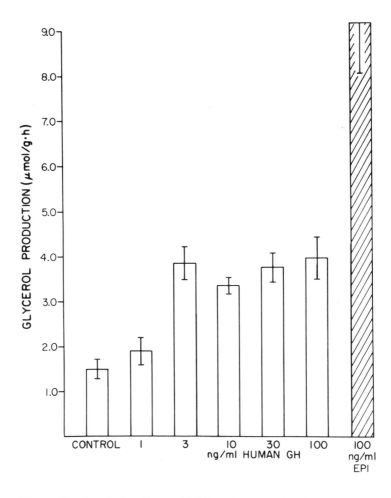

Figure 5.   Lipolytic effects of hGH and epinephrine in segments of adipose tissue in the fourth hour of incubation. Segments of adipose tissue from normal rats preincubated for 3 hours with 100 ng/ml of dexamethasone and the indicated concentrations of hGH. Epinephrine was present only in the fourth hour. Each bar represents the mean of eight observations. The standard errors are indicated by the vertical brackets. The effects of hGH were statistically significant at 3 ng/ml and above. The response to epinephrine was significantly greater than the response to the maximum concentration of hGH.

sponding to the low end of the range normally found in rat blood (55) significantly increased lipolysis in vitro.

In many experiments the dose–response relationship is more compressed than shown in Figure 4. In the experiment illustrated in Figure 5, the maximum lipolytic response seen in the fourth hour of incubation was produced in the presence of dexamethasone by hGH at a concentration of only 3 ng/ml. The 2.5-fold increase in glycerol production is typical of the magnitude of lipolysis produced by GH and dexamethasone. It is evident, however, that the rate of lipolysis produced by a saturating concentration of GH is small compared to the response that can be elicited by epinephrine in otherwise untreated tissues in the fourth hour of incubation. The lipolytic response to GH thus differs from that of epinephrine in both magnitude and rapidity of onset. Despite these differences, however, there is no reason to believe that GH and dexamethasone increase glycerol release by any other process than the cAMP-mediated pathway illustrated in Figure 1. The analogous cAMP-dependent process, activation of glycogen phosphorylase, is also stimulated by dexamethasone and GH (56,57), and with an identical time course. In addition, these hormones increased the concentration of cAMP in adipocyte cytosol in the fourth hour (58).

In the same range of concentrations, hGH also increased lipolysis in adipose tissue of hypophysectomized or normal rats when tested in the presence of the methylxanthine theophylline instead of glucocorticoids (Figure 6). Theophylline, which alone increases lipolysis, was originally thought to act by inhibiting cAMP phosphodiesterase (59, 60), thereby allowing cAMP formed by the basal activity of adenylate cyclase to accumulate. It now appears likely that the lipolytic activity of theophylline also results from its interaction with the adenosine receptor to block the inhibitory input of endogenous adenosine (61). A lag period of more than 1 hour is required for the effects of GH and theophylline to be demonstrable, and as with dexamethasone, 3 or 4 hours are needed for the full-blown response to develop. To obtain the data shown in Figure 6, segments of adipose tissue excised from hypophysectomized rats were preincubated for 3 hours with concentrations of GH ranging from 1 to 300 ng/ml and then transferred to fresh incubation medium for a final hour of incubation in the presence of 0.3 mg/ml of theophylline. In this experiment the minimal effective con-

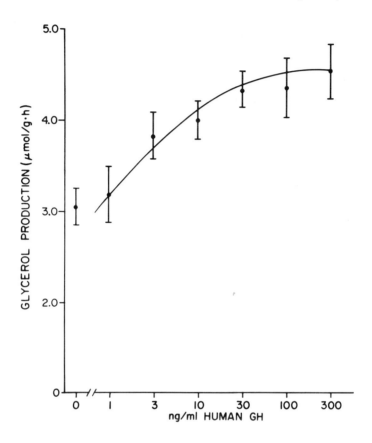

Figure 6.   Lipolytic effects of hGH in the presence of theophylline. Segments of epididymal adipose tissue from hypophysectomized rats were preincubated for 3 hours in the presence of 0–300 ng/ml of hGH and were then transferred to fresh medium for a final hour of incubation in the presence of 0.3 mg/ml of theophylline. Each point is the mean of eight observations, and the standard errors are indicated by the vertical brackets. The effects of GH were statistically significant at 3 ng/ml and above as determined by Duncan's multiple range test after two-way analysis of variance.

centration of hGH was 3 ng/ml, although in many experiments 1 ng/ml is sufficient. Once again, a maximum response was obtained with about 30 ng/ml and falls far short of the maximum capacity of the tissues for lipolysis.

In general, adipose tissue from hypophysectomized rats exhibits little or no response to GH and dexamethasone unless an agent such as theophylline is also present, or unless the hypophysectomized rats are pretreated with growth hormone prior to sacrifice (62). Figure 7 shows the total glycerol and FFA released by segments of adipose tissue incubated for 4 hours either without hormones or in the presence of dexamethasone and GH. These hormones increased the production of glycerol by normal tissues and by tissues of hypophysectomized rats that had been pretreated with GH, but they had little effect on tissues of untreated hypophysectomized animals. These results suggest that, in addition to its acute effects on lipolysis, GH may be necessary for chronic maintenance of the lipolytic system. This experiment also illustrates another point. Since 3 mol of fatty acid are liberated for every mole of glycerol released, it is evident that in tissues of both normal and hypophysectomized rats, the vast majority of fatty acids produced by lipolysis are reesterified. In fact, in the tissues of un-treated hypophysectomized animals, there was net uptake of the fatty acids which were introduced into the medium bound to albumin. GH and dexamethasone increased the ratio of fatty acids released to glycerol released, indicative of an inhibition of reesterification and an action of these hormones to increase the efficiency of lipolysis with respect to fatty acid mobilization.

Although we can find ways to rationalize its acting only after a long lag period, and even its having only a limited range of efficacy, it is difficult to understand how GH can serve as an initiator of lipolysis when the maximal response is produced by concentrations that are almost always present in blood. These considerations, and the observa-tions in vivo that the lipolytic effects of GH are most readily demon-strable when some other impetus for lipolysis, such as fasting, is also present (3), suggest that GH may function not as an agonist to initiate the lipolytic process, but rather as a modulator or amplifier of re-sponses to other hormones or endogenous signals. The results of the next experiment are consistent with this idea.

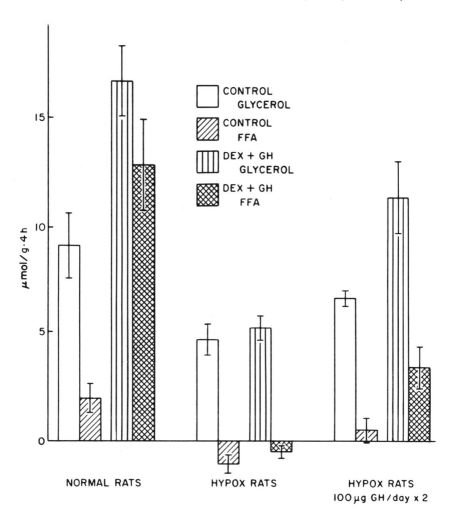

Figure 7. The effect of hypophysectomy and pretreatment with GH on the response to dexamethasone and GH added in vitro. The dexamethasone was present at a concentration of 0.16 μg/ml and the ovine GH at 1μg/ml. The tissues were incubated without transfer for 4 hours. The vertical bars represent the means of eight observations, and the vertical brackets indicate the standard errors. Dexamethasone and GH significantly increased both glycerol and FFA production in tissues of normal rats and hypophysectomized rats that had been pretreated with GH. (From Ref. 62.)

To test the hypothesis that GH might augment the response to another lipolytic signal, pairs of tissues obtained from hypophysectomized rats were preincubated for 3 hours without hormone, with dexamethasone alone, with GH alone, or with the combination of dexamethasone and GH (Figure 8). The tissues were then transferred to fresh medium for the final hour of incubation, with one tissue of each pair exposed to 10 ng/ml of epinephrine in the final incubation. The increase in glycerol production caused by epinephrine in each case is plotted. Preincubation with dexamethasone alone nearly tripled the amount of glycerol released in response to epinephrine. Preincubation with GH alone had no effect on the response to epinephrine, but epinephrine elicited the production of significantly more glycerol when tissues of hypophysectomized rats were preincubated with the combination of GH and dexamethasone than when preincubated with dexamethasone alone. Thus GH amplified the lipolytic response to epinephrine, but only in the presence of glucocorticoid. Similar results were obtained with isolated adipocytes (63) and tissues of normal rats (64).

To obtain some understanding of where GH might act in the lipolytic sequence, the previous experiment was repeated using the dibutyryl analog of cAMP instead of epinephrine as the lipolytic agonist (Figure 9). If the amplification caused by GH and dexamethasone is exerted at a step subsequent to the involvement of the cyclic nucleotide, an enhancement of lipolysis should be observed. If, on the other hand, the site of intervention of GH and dexamethasone is on some reaction earlier than the involvement of the cyclic nucleotide, there should be no enhancement of lipolysis. This indeed appeared to be the case. Neither GH nor dexamethasone, alone or in combination, increased the lipolytic action of a submaximal concentration of dibutyryl cAMP. Once again, pairs of tissue were incubated with GH and dexamethasone for the 3 hours preceding the addition of the lipolytic agent, and the data shown indicate the increase in glycerol produced in response to the cyclic nucleotide. Similar results were obtained by Fain using adipocytes from intact rats (63). These results suggest that both GH and dexamethasone produce their enhancing effects on lipolysis at a site early in the lipolytic sequence.

It has become almost axiomatic in endocrinology that when a

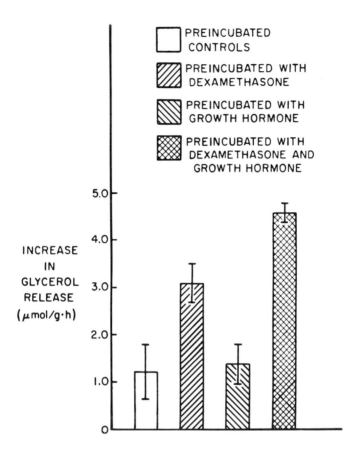

Figure 8. The effects of preincubation for 3 hours with dexamethasone and GH on subsequent lipolysis by tissues of hypophysectomized rats in response to 0.01 μg/ml of epinephrine. To obtain the effects of epinephrine under each experimental condition, pairs of tissues from nine rats were preincubated for 3 hours in the presence of dexamethasone (0.16 μg/ml), GH (1 μg/ml), both, or neither. The tissues were then transferred to fresh medium for the final hour of incubation, with one tissue of each pair exposed to epinephrine. Each bar represents the increment in glycerol production, with the vertical brackets indicating the standard errors. Dexamethasone alone significantly ($p < .01$) increased the response to epinephrine, and the combination of GH and dexamethasone produced a significantly ($p < .01$) greater response. (From Ref. 79.)

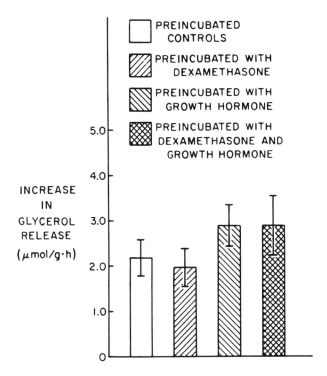

Figure 9. The effects of preincubation for 3 hours with dexamethasone and GH on subsequent lipolytic response of adipose tissue from hypophysectomized rats to 10^{-3} M dibutyryl cAMP. The experiment was designed as described for Figure 8. No significant increase in lipolysis resulted from any treatment. (From Ref. 80.)

latent period is required for the expression of a hormonal response a change in genetic expression should be expected. The delay that precedes the onset of the lipolytic response to GH thus has been attributed to the time needed for the induction of new proteins. Indeed, the findings that the increase in glycerol and fatty acids produced by dexamethasone and GH could be prevented with inhibitors of RNA and protein synthesis (65–67) suggested that expression of the lipolytic response required gene transcription and translation. However, the stimulation of lipolysis produced by GH in the presence of theophyl-

line requires the same delay as that required by GH and dexamethasone, even though it is not blocked by inhibitors of RNA and protein
synthesis (32). It is possible that the synthesis of new protein is needed
for action of dexamethasone, rather than GH, or that GH increases
lipolysis by at least two different routes, one of which requires altered
genetic expression and one of which does not. The delay in the expression of the effects of GH could result from the time needed for the
decay of some cellular constituent or the gradual attainment of a new
steady state when a small change is produced in the rate of only one of
a pair of opposing reactions.

While the preceding experiments are consistent with the hypothesis that GH enhances the ability of adipocytes to generate cyclic
nucleotides in response to lipolytic agonists, they do not provide convincing evidence that such an action is involved in the lipolytic effects
seen in the absence of agonists such as epinephrine. As already discussed, however, adenylate cyclase is under inhibitory as well as excitatory control. Prostaglandins and adenosine generated from endogenous sources appear to maintain adenylate cyclase at its low basal state
of activation in the absence of exogenous excitatory stimuli. Modulation of lipolysis by GH and dexamethasone could be achieved in the
absence of a stimulatory agonist if these hormones interfered with
either the production or action of endogenous inhibitors.

Prostaglandins are synthesized from arachidonic acid, which is
stored in membrane phospholipids and released by the action of an
enzyme, phospholipase A_2, so named because it cleaves the ester bond
at the 2 carbon of glycerol (68). Conversion of arachidonate to prostaglandin is catalyzed by cyclooxygenase, which appears to be present
in virtually all tissues (69). Mounting evidence suggests that glucocorticoids induce many cells to synthesize a protein inhibitor of phospholipase A_2, called macrocortin (70,71) or lipomodulin (72). By
inhibiting phospholipase A_2 activity, macrocortin, and hence glucocorticoids, blocks prostaglandin synthesis by depriving the cyclooxygenase enzyme system of substrate. The so-called nonsteroidal antiinflammatory agents such as aspirin and indomethacin also block
prostaglandin formation, but they produce their pharmacological effects by inhibiting cyclooxygenase (73,74).

The experiment seen in Figure 10 was designed to evaluate the

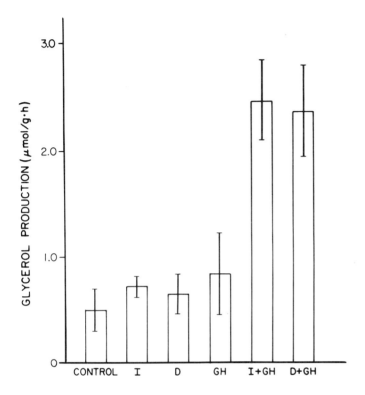

Figure 10. Lipolytic effects of GH in the presence of indomethacin or dexamethasone. Segments of adipose tissue from normal rats were preincubated for 3 hours with 50 μg/ml of indomethacin (I), 100 ng/ml of dexamethasone (D), 100 ng/ml of GH, or GH in combination with dexamethasone or indomethacin. The tissues were then transferred to fresh medium, and glycerol released in the final hour was assessed. Each bar represents the mean of eight observations, with the vertical brackets indicating the standard errors. Lipolysis was significantly ($p < .01$) increased in those tissues that preincubated with GH and indomethacin or GH and dexamethasone.

possibility that dexamethasone might potentiate the lipolytic effects of GH by inhibiting prostaglandin formation. Segments of adipose tissue were preincubated for 3 hours with dexamethasone, indomethacin, or GH, or the combination of GH and dexamethasone or GH and indomethacin. Tissues were then transferred to fresh medium and glycerol produced in the fourth hour was measured. When present alone, neither dexamethasone nor indomethacin produced any significant increase in glycerol production. However, both agents synergized with GH to produce the typical lipolytic response. Indomethacin was as effective as dexamethasone. Since the only other action that these two agents are known to share is antagonism of prostaglandin formation, it is likely that interference with the production of prostaglandin formation enables the lipolytic effects of GH to be observed. Furthermore, the apparent involvement of macrocortin could account for the sensitivity of the lipolytic effect of dexamethasone and GH to inhibitors of RNA and protein synthesis.

Elimination of the other major endogenous inhibitor, adenosine, by inclusion of adenosine deaminase in the incubation medium produced similar results, particularly when isolated adipocytes are studied instead of tissue segments (Figure 11). Once again the data shown represent the rates of glycerol released into the incubation medium during the fourth hour. Preincubation with GH alone for 3 hours produced little effect on lipolysis. Adenosine deaminase alone significantly increased glycerol production, and when combined with GH it enabled a lipolytic response of GH to become evident. These observations are highly reminiscent of our earlier findings with theophylline (32), which is thought to block the adenosine receptor (43,61).

It thus appears that decreasing the influence of inhibitory agonists is necessary for the lipolytic action of GH to be expressed. From the earlier studies with epinephrine and dibutyryl cAMP (Figures 8 and 9), it appeared that GH must act at a point in the lipolytic sequence that precedes the appearance of cAMP. Furthermore, the slowness in development and the limited magnitude of the response indicated that GH must act in some manner that is different from that of epinephrine. These considerations led us to examine the possibility that either or both of the guanine nucleotide binding proteins, N_s and N_i, might be targets of GH action.

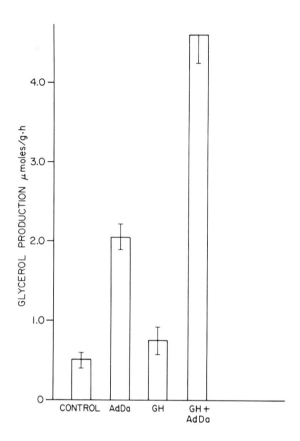

Figure 11. Lipolytic effects of GH in the presence of adenosine deaminase. Adipocytes obtained from normal rats were preincubated for 3 hours with 0.1 μU/ml adenosine deaminase (AdDa), 30 ng/ml hGH, or GH plus AdDa. The medium was then removed by aspiration and replaced with fresh medium for the assessment of glycerol production in the fourth hour of incubation. Each bar represents the mean of five replicate incubations, with the vertical brackets showing the standard errors. The response to the combination of GH and adenosine deaminase was greater than that produced by adenosine deaminase alone.

The inhibitory effects of adenosine and the prostaglandins are thought to be mediated by activation of the inhibitory guanine nucleotide binding protein, N_i, which couples their individual receptors to adenylate cyclase. N_i, which appears to be abundant in the adipocyte membrane, is comprised of three subunits, α, β, and γ (41–43). The 40,000-dalton α subunit appears to be the target of the toxin produced by the bacterium *Bortedelle pertussis* (75,76). Pertussis toxin contains an enzyme that catalyzes the transfer of the ADP-ribose component of NAD to an asparagine moiety of the α subunit of N_i to form an N-glycoside linkage. ADP ribosylation of N_i produces irreversible inactivation, and hence relieves the inhibition on adenylate cyclase. Incubation of adipose tissue or isolated human or rat adipocytes with pertussis toxin results in the gradual activation of lipolysis, which approaches the maximal capacity of the tissue by the fourth hour, supporting the suggestion that in the absence of exogenous agonists, the activity of adenylate cyclase is suppressed by endogenous inhibitory influences.

Stimulation of adenylate cyclase by epinephrine and other rapidly acting agonists is mediated by N_s, which is also comprised of three subunits designated α, β, and γ (41–43). The 45,000-dalton α subunit is the target of cholera toxin, which catalyzes the transfer of ADP-ribose from NAD to the guanidinium group of an arginine residue (76). ADP ribosylation of the α subunit of N_s blocks its ability to hydrolyze GTP (41), rendering it, and consequently adenylate cyclase, permanently active.

We have taken advantage of the actions of bacterial toxins to ADP ribosylate N_i or N_s specifically to study the effects of GH on these regulatory proteins, and some of our preliminary findings are presented here. Adipocyte ghosts were incubated with ^{32}P-labeled NAD of high specific radioactivity along with either cholera toxin or pertussis toxin under conditions that optimized protein ribosylation. Adipocyte ghosts were used instead of intact fat cells or segments of adipose tissue because of the impermeability of the cell membranes to NAD. At the end of the incubation period, the adipocyte ghosts were dissolved in SDS, and the proteins separated by electrophoresis on polyacrylamide gels. Autoradiographs were prepared, and the intensity of labeling of

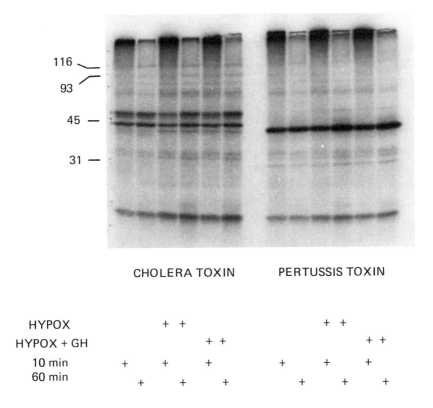

CHOLERA TOXIN   PERTUSSIS TOXIN

HYPOX	+	+		+	+	
HYPOX + GH			+ +			+ +
10 min	+	+	+	+	+	+
60 min		+	+	+	+	+	+

Figure 12. Autoradiograph from a one-dimensional SDS slab gel of the proteins of adipocyte ghosts labeled by incubation with cholera and pertussis toxins and [^{32}P]NAD$^+$. Ghosts were prepared from adipose tissues from six normal, six hypophysectomized (HYPOX), and six hypophysectomized rats treated with a single injection of 100 μg/rat 4 hours before sacrifice. Equal amounts of protein were incubated in the presence of cholera toxin or pertussis toxin and [^{32}P]NAD$^+$ for 10 or 60 minutes. The labeled proteins were separated by SDS-gel electrophoresis with slab gels of 10% polyacrylamide. The position of molecular weight standards is indicated at the left. Cholera toxin catalyzed the ribosylation of two major bands corresponding to M_r of 45,000 and 53,000. The 45,000-dalton band was presumed to be N$_{s\alpha}$. Pertussis toxin catalyzed the ribosylation of protein with M_r of 40,000-daltons presumed to be N$_{i\alpha}$.

specific protein bands was quantitated by densitometric scanning of the x-ray films.

The pattern of incorporation of [^{32}P]ADP-ribose into proteins of adipocyte ghosts is shown in Figure 12. Incubation with cholera toxin resulting in the labeling of two protein bands corresponding to molecular weights of 45 and 55 KD, while incubation with pertussis toxin resulted in the labeling of a band corresponding to M_r 40,000. Cholera toxin produced similar amounts of ADP ribosylation in adipocyte ghosts obtained from normal and hypophysectomized rats, and treatment of the hypophysectomized rats with 100 μg of GH 4 hours before sacrifice produced little or no effect. Cholera toxin–catalyzed ribosylation of N_s was essentially complete within 10 minutes of incubation, and further addition of either toxin or ^{32}P NAD failed to yield further ribosylation. In contrast, adipocyte ghosts prepared from the epididymal fat of hypophysectomized rats appeared to incorporate more labeled ADP-ribose into N_i than ghosts of normal fat cells, and the pretreatment with GH appeared to reduce ADP ribosylation of N_i. Ribosylation of N_i did not reach maximum until at least 1 hour, and was not increased by the further addition of ^{32}P NAD or pertussis toxin. Since these experiments were performed under conditions in which N_s or N_i was limiting, a change in the amount of ^{32}P incorporation is likely to indicate a change in either the amount or configuration of the N protein.

Figure 13 shows the densitometer scans of the 40–50 KD range of the autoradiogram shown in the previous slide. The numbers given above the main peaks represent the areas under the curves in arbitrary units of density. There can be little doubt that hypophysectomy increased the incorporation of ^{32}P into N_i, and GH appeared to decrease ribosylation of N_i. Table 1 summarizes our initial ribosylation experiments with either cholera toxin or pertussis toxin. To date we have found no consistent differences in the ribosylation of N_s by cholera toxin in adipocyte ghosts prepared from normal and hypophysectomized rats. Ribosylation of N_i by pertussis toxin in adipocyte ghosts prepared from hypophysectomized rats is markedly greater than that seen in ghosts from normal rats.

Because the effects of GH on the ribosylation of N_i and N_s are relatively modest, we modified our protocol to enable us to assess ribosylation of N_s and N_i in aliquots of the same preparation of adipo-

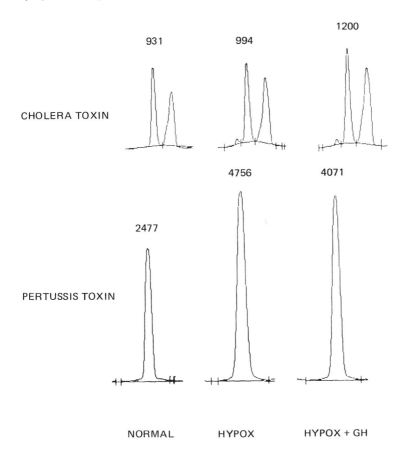

Figure 13. Optical density scans of cholera toxin and pertussis toxin labeled proteins in the 60-minute reactions shown in the autoradiograph in Figure 12. The output of the densitometer was digitized, and areas calculated by computer integration are expressed in arbitrary units above the 45,000-dalton (cholera toxin) and 40,000-dalton (pertussis toxin) peaks.

Table 1.   Effects of Growth Hormone on
^{32}P-NAD Ribosylation of N_s (cholera toxin) and
N_i (pertussis toxin) in Adipocyte Ghosts

	Density of ^{32}P-labeled protein band in arbitrary units	
	Normal	Hypox
	Cholera toxin	
	4,689	3,514
	4,141	2,311
	8,053	9,328
	2,371	2,441
	2,656	2,023
	9,126	13,205
	931	994
Mean	4,567	4,831
	Pertussis toxin	
	3,277	3,970
	5,200	8,878
	4,503	10,822
	2,002	2,952
	2,005	3,839
	2,477	4,757
Mean	3,244	5,870

cyte ghosts (Table 2). In three separate experiments, adipocyte ghosts
prepared from hypophysectomized rats which had received an intraperitoneal injection of 100 μg of GH 3 hours before sacrifice exhibited
less pertussis toxin–dependent ribosylation than ghosts from control
animals. It is likely that the stoichiometry of the N proteins determines
the balance between inhibitory and stimulatory influences on adenylate
cyclase. When the data are expressed in terms of the ratio of ^{32}P in the
two regulatory proteins, it appears that GH may tip the balance toward

Table 2. Effects of Growth Hormone on ^{32}P-NAD Ribosylation of N_s (cholera toxin) and N_i (pertussis toxin) in Adipocyte Ghosts

Experiment	Density of ^{32}P-labeled protein band in arbitrary units			
	Hypox	PT/CT	Hypox + GH	PT/CT
	Cholera toxin			
1	3910		4009	
2	2350		2600	
3	514		657	
Mean	2258		2422	
	Pertussis toxin			
1	8319	2.13	6217	1.55
2	4620	1.97	4150	1.60
3	1450	2.82	1294	1.97
Mean	4796	2.31	3887	1.71

stimulation, consistent with the proposition that N_i may be a target of GH action.

To verify that a change in N_i can indeed increase lipolysis in segments of adipose tissue, we preincubated tissues for 3 hours in our usual manner with various concentrations of pertussis toxin. The tissues were then transferred to fresh incubation medium to permit measurement of glycerol release during the fourth hour (Figure 14). This protocol was followed both to examine pertussis toxin under the same conditions used for GH and dexamethasone and because studies on the effects of the toxin in adipocytes indicated that the response to pertussis is slow in onset (77) with a time course resembling that of GH.

If we pursue the suggestion that N_i may be modified either in amount or configuration by GH, our earlier model of the regulation of adenylate cyclase in adipose tissue can be revised as illustrated in Figure 15. Adenylate cyclase activity appears to be determined by the

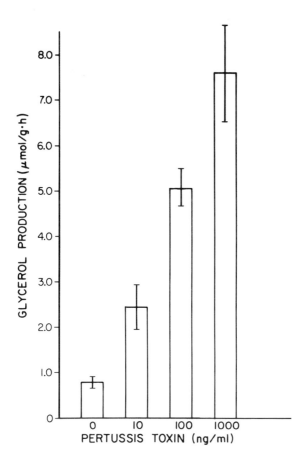

Figure 14. The effects of pertussis toxin on glycerol production by segments of epididymal adipose tissue obtained from normal rats. The tissues were preincubated for 3 hours with 0–1000 ng/ml of pertussis toxin, and then transferred to fresh medium for assessment of glycerol production in the fourth hour of incubation. Each bar represents the mean of eight observations, with the vertical brackets indicating the standard errors. The toxin significantly ($p < .01$) increased lipolysis at all concentrations tested.

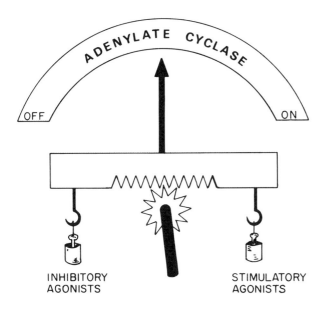

Figure 15. Interaction of stimulatory and inhibitory factors on the activity of adenyl cyclase. Modulation of the input of stimulatory and inhibitory factors, accomplished by the activity of N_s or N_i, is represented by the movable fulcrum. An action of GH to decrease the influence of N_i would be equivalent to turning the crank handle to the left. An action of dexamethasone to decrease prostaglandin synthesis would be equivalent to removing some of the weight on the left side of the lever arm. An action of theophylline to block adenosine receptors or adenosine deaminase to decrease extracellular adenosine would similarly be equivalent to removing some of the weight on the left side of the lever arm. The possibility of an interaction between adenosine and prostaglandin to regulate each other's production has not been studied.

balance between stimulatory and inhibitory agonists as shown in Figure 2, but because the efficacy of coupling of the input with adenylate cyclase may be subject to regulation by the action of GH, a given amount of stimulatory or inhibitory input may not always produce the same stimulation or inhibition. This is represented in the figure by balancing the stimulatory and inhibitory inputs on a movable fulcrum. It appears from our results with indomethacin that dexamethasone may affect lipolysis by inhibiting prostaglandin formation and thus decreasing the inhibitory force exerted on the lever arm. By decreasing the availability of N_i, GH, in effect, turns the crank handle to the left, foreshortening the length of the lever arm bearing the inhibitory agonist. Therefore, even if the downward pull of inhibitory agonists remained relatively constant, the degree of inhibition felt by the enzyme would be reduced, and thus produce a small increase in lipolysis, as is seen in some experiments. When the inhibitory input of the prostaglandins is simultaneously reduced by dexamethasone, or that of adenosine by theophylline, the effect of GH is magnified, and an increase in lipolysis becomes evident. It will be of particular interest to learn if the production of prostaglandins and the production of adenosine are in any way mutually interdependent. This model appears to be consistent with most of the available information on the lipolytic effects of GH and provides a conceptual framework for addressing the question of how GH might modulate lipolysis without serving as a primary agonist.

The concept that adenylate cyclase is under the inhibitory control of endogenous paracrine factors as well as stimulatory hormones provides a new approach for the understanding of permissive actions of glucocorticoids and of thyroxine as well as GH. Any of these hormones might regulate the formation of inhibitory agonists or act by modifying N_i or N_s. Certainly the observation that there is an apparent increase in N_i in adipose tissue after hypophysectomy is consistent with our earlier findings that tissues of hypophysectomized animals show a considerable decrease in sensitivity to stimulation by lipolytic agents (78). Finally, sufficient information on the molecular actions of many hormones is now available to suggest that it may be naive to expect that hormonal effects as complex as those of GH are limited to a single locus of action. The putative action on N_i may thus represent only part of the explanation of how GH increases lipolysis.

ACKNOWLEDGMENTS

Various preparations of GH have been generously supplied by the National Pituitary Agency, Genentech Incorporated, Kabi Vitrium, Dr. Jack L. Kostyo, and Dr. U. J. Lewis. The authors are particularly indebted to Mrs. L. R. Tai, Mr. L. R. Waice, and Dr. L. K. Levy for their superb efforts in support of these studies.

REFERENCES

1. Lee MO, Shaeffer NK. Anterior pituitary growth hormone and the composition of growth. J. Nutr. 7:337–363, 1934.

2. Astwood EB. Growth hormone and corticotropin. In The Hormones, vol. 3, Pincus G, Thimann K, eds., Academic Press, New York, 1955, pp. 235–308.

3. Goodman HM, Schwartz J. Growth hormone and lipid metabolism. In Handbook of Physiology: Endocrinology, Part 2, Knobil E, Sawyer W, eds., The American Physiological Society, Washington, 1974, pp. 211–231.

4. DeBodo RC, Altszuler N. The metabolic effects of growth hormone and their physiological significance. Vitamins and Hormones 15:205–258, 1957.

5. Ketterer B, Randle PJ, Young FG. The pituitary growth hormone and metabolic processes. Ergeb. Physiol. Biol. Chem. Exp. Pharmakol. 49:127–211, 1957.

6. Weil R. Metabolic function of the pituitary growth hormone. Arch. Int. Med. 95:739–760, 1955.

7. Barrett HM, Best CH, Ridout JH. A study of the source of liver fat using deuterium as an indicator. J. Physiol. 93:367–381, 1938.

8. Stetten DN Jr, Salcedo J Jr. The source of extra liver fat in various types of fatty liver. J. Biol. Chem. 156:27–32, 1944.

9. Li CH, Evans HM, Simpson ME. Isolation and properties of the anterior hypophyseal growth hormone. J. Biol. Chem. 159:353–366, 1945.

10. Wilhelmi AE, Fishman JB, Russell JA. A new preparation of crystalline anterior pituitary growth hormone. J. Biol. Chem. 176:735–746, 1948.

11. Beaton GH, Curry DM. A comparison of the effects of growth hormone and insulin administration. Endocrinology 58:797–801, 1956.

12. Greenbaum AL. Changes in body composition and respiratory quotient of normal female rats treated with purified growth hormone. Biochem. J. 54:400–407, 1953.

13. Li CH, Simpson ME, Evans HM. Gigantism produced in normal rats produced by injection of the pituitary growth hormone. III. Main chemical components of the body. Growth 12:39–42, 1948.

14. Li CH, Simpson ME, Evans HM. Influence of growth and adrenocorticotropic hormones on the body composition of hypophysectomized rats. Endocrinology 44:71–75, 1949.

15. Tanner JM, Whitehouse RH. The effect of human growth hormone on subcutaneous fat thickness in hyposomatotrophic and panhypopituitary dwarfs. J. Endocrinol. 39:263–275, 1967.

16. Bonnet F, Vanderschueren-Lodewyck X, Eekels R, Malvaux P. Subcutaneous adipose tissue and lipids in blood in growth hormone deficiency before and after treatment with human growth hormone. Pediat. Res. 8:800–805, 1974.

17. Dole VP. A relation between non-esterified fatty acids in plasma and metabolism of glucose. J. Clin. Invest. 35:206–212, 1956.

18. Gordon RS, Cherkes A. Unesterified fatty acids in human blood plasma. J. Clin. Invest. 35:206–212, 1956.

19. Raben MS, Hollenberg CH. Effects of growth hormone on plasma fatty acids. J. Clin. Invest. 38:484–488, 1959.

20. Engel HR, Hellman L, Siegal S, Bergenstal DM. Effect of growth hormone on plasma unesterified fatty acid levels of hypophysectomized rats. Proc. Soc. Exp. Biol. Med. 98:753–755, 1958.

21. Goodman HM, Knobil E. Growth hormone and fatty acid mobilization: The role of the pituitary, adrenal and thyroid. Endocrinology 69:187–189, 1961.

22. Knobil E. Direct evidence for fatty acid mobilization in response to growth hormone administration in the rat. Proc. Soc. Exp. Biol. Med. 101:288–289, 1959.

23. Kovacev VP, Scow RO. Effect of hormones on fatty acid release by adipose tissue in vivo. Am. J. Physiol. 210:1199–1208, 1966.

24. Swislocki NI, Szego CM. Acute reduction of plasma non-esterified fatty acids by growth hormone in hypophysectomized and Houssay rats. Endocrinology 76:655–672, 1965.

25. Beck JC, McGarry EE, Dyrenfurth I, Morgen RO, Bird E, Venning EH. The variability in physiological response to growth hormone. Ciba Foundation Colloquia in Endocrinology 13:156–173, 1960.

26. Engel HR, Bergenstal DM, Nixon WE, Patten JA. Effect of human growth hormone on unesterified fatty acids and plasma amino nitrogen in man. Proc. Soc. Exp. Biol. Med. 100:699–701, 1958.

27. Henneman DH, Henneman PH. Effects of human growth hormone on levels of blood and urinary carbohydrate and fat metabolites in man. J. Clin. Invest. 39:1239–1245, 1960.

28. Goodman HM, Knobil E. Effects of fasting and of growth hormone on plasma fatty acid concentration in normal and hypophysectomized rhesus monkeys. Endocrinology 65:451–458, 1959.

29. Gerich JE, Lorenzi M, Bier DM, Tsalikian E, Schneider V, Karam JH, Forsham PH. Effects of physiological levels of glucagon and growth hormone on human carbohydrate and lipid metabolism. J. Clin. Invest. 57:875–884, 1976.

30. Scow RO, Chernick SS. Mobilization, transport, and utilization of free fatty acids. In Comprehensive Biochemistry, vol. 18, Lipid Metabolism, Florkin M, Stutz EH, eds., Elsevier, Amsterdam, 1970, pp. 20–50.

31. Fain JN, Kovacev VP, Scow RO. Effect of growth hormone and dexamethasone on lipolysis and metabolism in isolated fat cells of the rat. J. Biol. Chem. 240:3522–3529, 1965.

32. Goodman HM. Effect of growth hormone on the lipolytic response of adipose tissue to theophylline. Endocrinology 82:1027–1034, 1968.

33. Goodman HM, Grichting G. Growth hormone and lipolysis: A reevaluation. Endocrinology 113:1111–1120, 1983.

34. Goodman HM. Biological activity of bacterial derived human growth hormone in adipose tissue of hypophysectomized rats. Endocrinology 114:131–135, 1984.

35. Steinberg D, Huttunen JK. The role of cyclic AMP in activation of hormone-sensitive lipase of adipose tissue. In Advances in Cyclic Nu-

cleotide Research, vol. 1, Greengard P, Paoletti R, Robison GA, eds., Raven Press, New York, 1972, pp. 47–62.

36. Steinberg D. Interconvertible enzymes in adipose tissue regulated by cyclic AMP-dependent protein kinase. In Advances in Cyclic Nucleotide Research, vol. 7, Greengard P, Robison GA, eds., Raven Press, New York, 1976, pp. 157–198.

37. Margolis S, Vaughan M. α-Glycerophosphate synthesis and breakdown in homogenates of adipose tissue. J. Biol. Chem. 237:44–48, 1962.

38. Goodman HM. Failure of growth hormone alone to potentiate epinephrine-induced lipolysis. Proc. Soc. Exp. Biol. Med. 132:821–824, 1967.

39. Goodman HM. Growth hormone and the metabolism of carbohydrate and lipid in adipose tissue. Ann. New York Acad. Sci. 148:419–440, 1968.

40. Stralfors P, Bjorgell P, Belfrage P. Hormonal regulation of hormone-sensitive lipase in intact adipocytes: Identification of phosphorylated sites and effects on the phosphorylation by lipolytic hormones and insulin. Proc. Natl. Acad. Sci. USA 81:3317–3321, 1984.

41. Birnbaumer L, Codina J, Mattera R, Cerione RA, Hildebrandt JD, Sunyer T, Rojas FJ, Caron MG, Lefkowitz RJ, Iyengar R. Regulation of hormone receptors and adenylyl cyclases by guanine nucleotide binding N proteins. Rec. Prog. Horm. Res. 41:41–94, 1985.

42. Gilman AG. G proteins and dual control of adenylate cyclase. Cell 36:577–579, 1984.

43. Cooper DMF, Londos C. GTP-dependent stimulation and inhibition of adenylate cyclase. In Horizons in Biochemistry and Biophysics, vol. 6, Hormone Receptors, Kohn LD, ed., Wiley-Interscience, New York, 1982, pp. 309–333.

44. Chang J, Lewis GP, Piper PJ. Inhibition by glucocorticoids of prostaglandin release from adipose tissue in vitro. Br. J. Pharmacol. 59:425–432, 1977.

45. Mitchell MD, Cleland WH, Smith ME, Simpson ER, Mendelson CR. Inhibition of prostaglandin biosynthesis in human adipose tissue by glucocorticosteroids. J. Clin. Endocrinol. Metab. 57:771–776, 1983.

46. Kather H, Bieger W, Michel G, Aktories K, Jakobs KH. Human fat cell

lipolysis is primarily regulated by inhibitory modulators acting through distinct mechanisms. J. Clin. Invest. 76:1559–1565, 1985.

47. Fain JN, Malbon CC. Regulation of adenylate cyclase by adenosine. Mol. Cell. Biochem. 25:143–169, 1979.

48. Schwabe UR, Ebert R, Erbler HG. Adenosine release from isolated fat cells and its significance for the effects of hormones on cyclic 3′,5′-AMP levels and lipolysis. Nauyn Schmiedebergs Arch. Pharmacol. 276:133–148, 1973.

49. Ohisalo JJ. Effects of adenosine on lipolysis in human subcutaneous fat cells. J. Clin. Endocrinol. Metab. 52:359–363, 1981.

50. Schecter Y. Evaluation of adenosine or related nucleosides as physiological regulators of lipolysis in adipose tissue. Endocrinology 110: 1579–1583, 1982.

51. Loten EG, Sneyd JGT. An effect of insulin on adipose tissue adenosine 3′,5′-monophosphate phosphodiesterase. Biochem. J. 120:187–193, 1970.

52. Senft G, Schultz G, Munske K, Hoffman M. Effects of glucocorticoids and insulin on 3′5′-AMP phosphodiesterase activity in adrenalectomized rats. Diabetologia 4:330–335, 1968.

53. Van Inwegen RG, Robison GA, Thompson WJ, Armstrong KJ, Stouffer JE. Cyclic nucleotide phosphodiesterases and thyroid hormones. J. Biol. Chem. 250:2452–2456, 1975.

54. Bilezikian JP, Loeb JN. The influence of hyperthyroidism and hypothyroidism on α- and β-adrenergic receptor systems and adrenergic responsiveness. Endocrine Rev. 4:378–388, 1983.

55. Tannenbaum GS, Martin JB, Colle E. Evidence for an endogenous ultradian rhythm governing growth hormone secretion in the rat. Endocrinology 99:720–727, 1976.

56. Eisen HG, Goodman HM. Growth hormone and phosphorylase activity in adipose tissue. Endocrinology 84:414–416, 1969.

57. Moskowitz J, Fain JN. Hormonal regulation of lipolysis and phosphorylase activity in human fat cells. J. Clin. Invest. 48:1802–1808, 1969.

58. Moskowitz J, Fain JN. Stimulation by growth hormone and dexametha-

sone of labeled cyclic adenosine 3′,5′-monophosphate accumulation by white fat cells. J. Biol. Chem. 245:1101–1107, 1970.

59. Butcher RW, Sutherland EW. Adenosine 3′,5′-phosphate in biological materials. I. Purification and properties of cyclic 3′,5′-nucleotide phosphodiesterase and use of this enzyme to characterize adenosine 3′,5′-phosphate in human urine. J. Biol. Chem. 237:1244–1250, 1962.

60. Butcher RW, Baird CE, Sutherland EW. Effects of lipolytic and antilipolytic substances on adenosine 3′,5′-phosphate levels in isolated fat cells. J. Biol. Chem. 243:1705–1712, 1968.

61. Londos C, Cooper DMF, Schlegel W, Rodbell M. Adenosine analogs inhibit adipocyte adenylate cyclase by a GTP-dependent process: Basis for action of adenosine and methylxanthines on cyclic AMP production and lipolysis. Proc. Natl. Acad. Sci. USA 75:5362–5366, 1978.

62. Goodman HM. Multiple effects of growth hormone on lipolysis. Endocrinology 83:300–308, 1968.

63. Fain JN. Effect of dibutyryl-3′,5′-AMP, theophylline and norepinephrine on lipolytic action of growth hormone and glucocorticoid on white fat cells. Endocrinology 82:825–830, 1968.

64. Goodman HM. The effects of epinephrine on glycerol production in segments of adipose tissue preincubated with dexamethasone and growth hormone. Proc. Soc. Exp. Biol. Med. 130:909–912, 1969.

65. Fain JN. Studies on the role of RNA and protein synthesis in the lipolytic action of growth hormone in isolated fat cells. Adv. Enzyme Reg. 5:39–51, 1967.

66. Fain JN, Saperstein R. Involvement of RNA synthesis and cyclic AMP in the activation of fat cell lipolysis by growth hormone and glucocorticoids. In Adipose Tissue, Regulation and Metabolic Functions, Jeanrenaud B, Hepp D, eds., Academic Press, New York, 1970, pp. 20–27.

67. Fain JN. Inhibition of lipolytic action of growth hormone and glucocorticoid by ultraviolet and x irradiation. Science 157:1062–1064, 1967.

68. Flower RJ, Blackwell GJ. The importance of phospholipase A in prostaglandin biosynthesis. Biochem. Pharmacol. 25:285–291, 1976.

69. Kuehl FA, Egan RW. Prostaglandins, arachidonic acid and inflammation. Science 210:978–984, 1980.

70. Flower RJ, Blackwell GJ. Antiinflammatory steroids induce biosynthesis of a phospholipase A_2 inhibitor which prevents prostaglandin generation. Nature 278:456–457, 1979.

71. Blackwell GF, Carnuccio R, DiRosa M, Flower RJ, Parente L, Persico P. Macrocortin: A polypeptide causing the antiphospholipase effects of glucocorticoids. Nature 287:147–148, 1980.

72. Hirata F. The regulation of lipomodilin, a phospholipase inhibitory protein in rabbit neutrophils by phosphorylation. J. Biol. Chem. 256:7730–7733, 1981.

73. Vane JR. Inhibition of prostaglandin synthesis as a mechanism of action for aspirin-like drugs. Nature (New Biol.):231:232–235, 1971.

74. Smith JB, Willis AL. Aspirin selectively inhibits prostaglandin production in human platelets. Nature (New Biol.):231:235–237, 1971.

75. Ui M, Nogimori K, Tamura M. Islet-activating protein, pertussis toxin: Subunit structure and mechanism for its multiple biological actions. In Pertussis Toxin, Sekura RD, Moss J, Vaughan M, eds., Academic Press, New York, 1985, pp. 19–44.

76. Ueda K, Hayaishi O. ADP-ribosylation. Ann. Rev. Biochem. 54:73–100, 1985.

77. Sekura RD, Zhang Y-I. Pertussis toxin: Structural elements involved in the interaction with cells. In Pertussis Toxin, Sekura RD, Moss J, Vaughan M, eds., Academic Press, New York, 1985, pp. 45–64.

78. Goodman HM. Endocrine control of lipolysis. In Progress in Endocrinology. Proceedings of the 3rd International Congress of Endocrinology, Mexico City, Gual C, ed. Excerpta Medica, Amsterdam, 1968, pp. 115–123.

79. Goodman HM. Permissive effects of hormones on lipolysis. Endocrinology 86:1064, 1970.

80. Goodman HM. Endocrine control of lipolysis. In Progress in Endocrinology: Proceedings of the Third International Congress of Endocrinology, Excerpta Medica Foundation, Amsterdam, 1969.

5

Neuroendocrine Regulation of Growth Hormone Secretion

MICHAEL O. THORNER and ALAN D. ROGOL

University of Virginia School of Medicine
Charlottesville, Virginia

Growth hormone is secreted in an intermittent pulsatile fashion during childhood and in adult life (1,2). It is therefore difficult to accept that GH secretion is important only for sustaining linear growth. There is evidence to suggest that GH is an important regulator of intermediary metabolism (3–5), and it probably plays a role in maintaining positive nitrogen balance, muscle mass, and bone density. In this chapter we briefly review the regulation of GH secretion and tests of GH reserve. The basis of these tests is discussed with special emphasis on their interpretation.

The complex nature of regulation of GH secretion is presented in Figure 1. Growth hormone is secreted by the somatotropes of the anterior pituitary under the influence of stimulatory and inhibitory

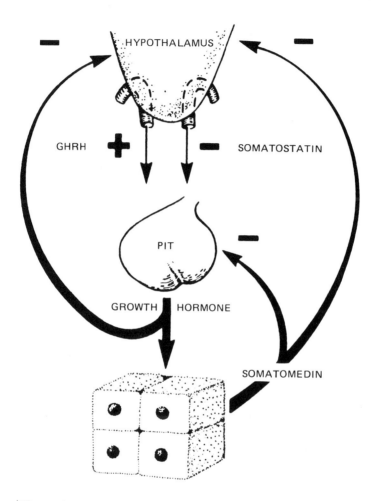

Figure 1.   Hypothalamic-growth hormone-somatomedin axis. Regulation of GH secretion. GH secretion by the pituitary is stimulated by GHRH and inhibited by somatostatin. Negative feedback control of the pituitary is exerted at the pituitary level by Sm-C. Somatomedin also acts on the hypothalamus to stimulate secretion of somatostatin. Based on indirect pharmacological data, it appears that release of GHRH is stimulated by actylcholine, α-adrenergic, and dopaminergic stimuli, and inhibited by β-adrenergic stimuli. Secretion of somatostatin, studied by direct assay in vitro, is stimulated by acetylcholine and vasoactive intestinal peptide and inhibited by GABA. Secretion of GH is modified by endogenous sleep rhythms, by stress, and by exercise. (From Ref. 6.)

factors. The somatotropes are regulated by two hypothalamic hormones, somatostatin (somatotropin release-inhibiting hormone, or SRIH) and growth hormone-releasing hormone (GHRH). In addition, somatomedin C [insulinlike growth factor I (IGF-I)] feeds back at both the pituitary and hypothalamic levels to inhibit GH secretion. GHRH and somatostatin are synthesized by neurons that have cell bodies lying within the hypothalamus. In turn, these neurons are regulated by monoaminergic and cholinergic neurons from other areas of the brain. The latter neurons act as transducers for environmental factors to regulate GH secretion. Factors that stimulate GH secretion include deep sleep, stress (physical and psychological), and exercise (6). In addition, nutrient intake modulates GH secretion in humans. Oral glucose loading suppresses GH secretion as blood glucose concentrations increase, but after 90–120 minutes GH secretion is stimulated when blood glucose concentrations decline (6). The change or rate of change in blood glucose therefore may be more important than the absolute concentration. Similarly, amino acids, particularly arginine and ornithine, stimulate GH secretion. The effects of mixed nutrients on GH secretion are variable and unpredictable (6).

In rats, GH is secreted rhythmically with an ultradian (fixed period over 24 hours) periodicity of approximately 3.3 hours (7). Although it has been thought that there is no such ultradian rhythm in humans, such rhythms may emerge in two situations. During puberty approximately eight pulses of GH occur every 24 hours (1). Normal young men who are fasted for 12–36 hours or longer manifest increased frequency of GH secretory events and increased basal and mean GH concentrations (Figure 2). Spectral analysis of these data demonstrate the emergence of several dominant frequencies, the most robust at one episode per 90 minutes (8). Thus a basic ultradian rhythm together with the effects of nutrients, exercise, sleep, and stress are all important considerations. The nutritional state of Western men may account for the apparent suppression of growth hormone secretion in adult life.

Growth hormone mediates many of its effects by stimulating the production of somatomedin C by the liver and many other tissues. Circulating Sm-C levels feed back at the hypothalamus and pituitary to inhibit GH secretion (Figure 1). However, Sm-C production (at least

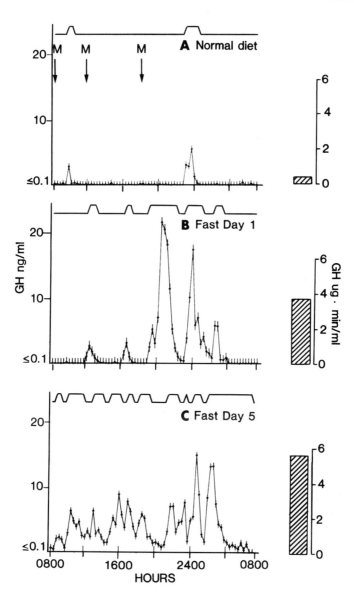

Figure 2. Serum GH levels measured every 20 minutes for 24 hours in a normal 37-year-old male prior to (A), during day 1 (B), and during day 5 (C) of a 5-day fast. Computer identification of GH pulses are shown above each profile. The shaded bars indicate integrated GH (μg minute/ml) of each of the 3 days. (From Ref. 24.)

by the liver) is regulated not only by the circulating concentration of GH but also by the nutritional state of the individual. For example, in protein-calorie malnutrition, Sm-C concentrations are low whereas GH concentrations are high. Nutritional rehabilitation of children results in a rapid increase in Sm-C levels, suppression of GH concentrations, and the initiation of accelerated growth (9) (Figure 3). It is possible therefore that the secretion of GH is regulated predominantly by the metabolic requirements of the individual, which in turn depend on the

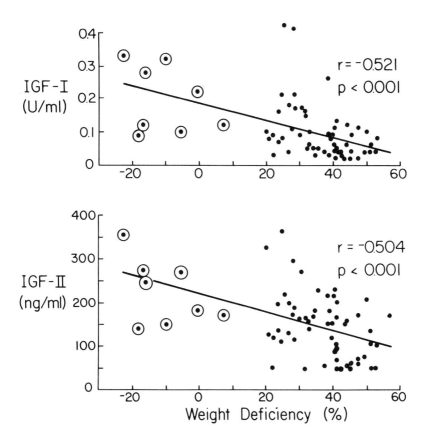

Figure 3. Serum insulinlike growth factor (IGF) concentrations and percent weight deficit in malnourished (●) and control children (⊙) before nutritional rehabilitation. (From Ref. 9.)

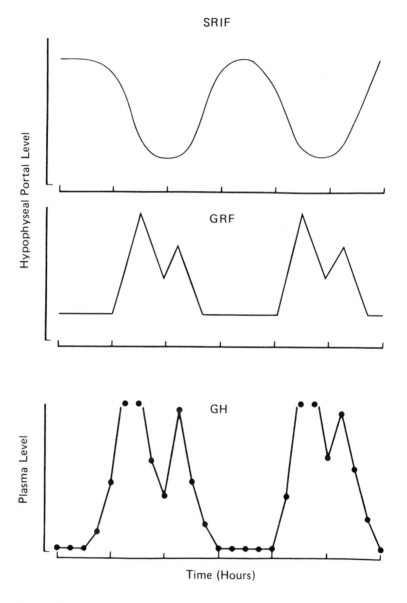

Figure 4. Schematic representation of the postulated rhythmic secretion of SRIF and GRF with the net result on GH secretion. (From Ref. 10.)

subject's nutritional state. Although this may be considered a non-hypothesis, there is much evidence to support it.

The pulsatile secretion of growth hormone is regulated by the reciprocal secretion of GHRH and somatostatin (10) (Figure 4). Evidence favoring this is derived from the demonstration of augmented pulsatile GH secretion in normal men during continuous (6 hour, 24 hour, and 14 day) infusions of GHRH, and pulsatile GH secretion in patients with persistently elevated GHRH levels due to ectopic secretion (11–13). In rats there is more direct evidence, since effects of endogenous somatostatin and GHRH can be blocked by passive immunization of the animal, permitting study of the effects of replacing GHRH and somatostatin (10). While the rat may be a good model for studying the pulsatile nature of GH secretion, it is probably not useful for understanding the effects of nutrients, gonadal steroids, and stress because these factors appear to have different effects in rat and man. These apparent paradoxes deserve further study.

Our understanding of the neurotransmitters regulating hypothalamic GHRH and somatostatin secretion is rudimentary (6). Experimental data support a role for α-adrenergic stimulation of GHRH secretion and β-adrenergic stimulation of somatostatin (14). In addition, cholinergic mechanisms may stimulate somatostatin secretion. In man, there is evidence of dopaminergic inhibition of somatostatin secretion. However, all the data are inferential.

I. GROWTH HORMONE SECRETION IN HUMANS

Growth hormone is secreted in pulses (bursts) at all stages of life. Recently we completed a study to define the precise pattern of GH secretion in young (18–30 years) and older (>55 years) men and women. Blood samples were withdrawn every 20 minutes for 24 hours for the determination of GH concentrations. The pulses of GH secretion were analyzed objectively using a statistically validated computer algorithm (2). We observed that women secrete more GH than men, and older men and women secrete less GH than young women. In Figure 5, representative profiles of GH secretion over 24 hours are shown from a young woman, young man, older woman, and older

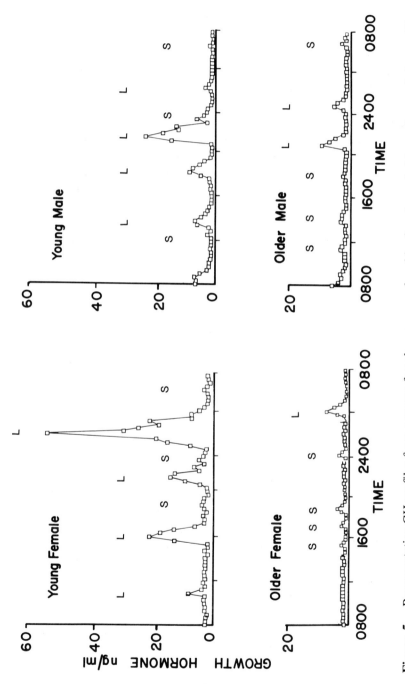

Figure 5. Representative GH profiles from a young female, young male, older female, and older male sampled every 20 minutes for 24 hours. Pulses were categorized as large (L) or small (S) depending on whether the rise was greater or less than three times the threshold criterion for a pulse. (From Ref. 2.)

man. In the young woman it is clear that the area under the curve is greater than in the older woman and older man. In addition, the number of pulses tends to be higher. These data are summarized for the entire group of volunteers in Table 1. Note that the integrated mean GH concentration is greater in young women than in young men and that young men, older women, and older men secrete roughly the same quantity of GH per day. The integrated GH concentrations correlate with the plasma estradiol concentrations (total or free), as do the amplitude of the pulses and the fraction of GH secreted as pulses. These data suggest that estradiol may be an important factor regulating GH secretion in humans. In contrast there was no correlation of GH with serum testosterone concentrations. The Sm-C level also correlated with the amount of growth hormone secreted in pulses ($r = .44$).

Growth hormone secretion and serum somatomedin C concentrations increase at puberty. This may be related to the rise in plasma estradiol both in boys and girls. However, GH and Sm-C concentrations normally rise before the first biochemical or clinical signs of puberty. The increase in GH and Sm-C could be related to the secretion of estrogens from the adrenal at adrenarche.

Testosterone treatment can increase GH secretion in children (15). Although the mechanism(s) for this is not known, it is possible that androgen may have been aromatized to estrogen. The increase in GH secretion at puberty represents an amplitude-modulated phenomenon

Table 1. Effects of Sex and Age on Pulsatile GH Secretion in Man

	Age	Integrated µg · min/ml	Pulses per 24 h		
			All	Small	Large
Young					
Women (13)	18–30	7.72	6.1	2.0	4.2
Men (7)	18–30	3.95	5.0	2.0	3.0
Older					
Women (8)	>55	3.37	3.7	2.5	1.1
Men (8)	>55	3.63	4.5	2.8	1.6

that is relatively independent of changes in pulse frequency. Such changes may be secondary to the action of sex steroid hormones modulating the responsivity of the somatotrope to endogenous GHRH, the amount of GHRH secreted, or the tonic inhibitory tone of somatostatin.

II. TESTS FOR GROWTH HORMONE RESERVE

Unfortunately, there are no absolutely reliable tests of GH reserve. Several different approaches have been taken. Because exercise and sleep are known stimuli of GH secretion, two simple tests are to have the patient exercise vigorously (e.g., run up and down several flights of stairs for 10 or 15 minutes and then measure serum GH at intervals for 20 minutes) and to measure serum GH after the patient has been asleep for 30–60 minutes in the hope of capturing the sleep-entrained rise in GH concentration. Both these tests have the advantage that they measure GH in response to physiological stimuli.

Because these tests frequently are inconclusive, others that utilize what are considered to be more reliable methods for stimulating GH secretion are employed. These tests include the induction of hypoglycemia with insulin, the infusion of L-arginine, and the administration of L-dopa orally. However, most investigators agree that none of these tests is entirely satisfactory since none is physiological. For all of these tests, a GH response above 7–10 ng/ml is traditionally considered to exclude GH deficiency. (Also see discussion of controversies in growth hormone therapy.)

Related questions include the following: What amount and pattern of GH secretion are necessary for normal growth? Is it the amount of GH secreted over a 24-hour period, the pattern (number of pulses), or the amplitude of pulses that is critical? The studies of Clark et al. (16) in rats demonstrate that if GH is administered continuously there is less effect on growth compared to the same amount given intermittently. Similar experiments have not been reported in humans. What is normal GH secretion and what criteria define GH deficiency? At the extremes of the spectrum, these answers are relatively easy. The child who grows normally, has parents of normal neight, and attains a normal adult height has sufficient GH, irrespective of the pattern of GH secretion. In contrast, the child who has a subnormal growth velocity, has fallen behind on cumulative height charts, and has no GH response to dynamic function tests has GH deficiency. The problem lies with the children who do not fall into these two extreme categories.

An alternative to provocative testing is to sample blood for GH at intervals of every 10 or 20 minutes over 24 hours. The results of such studies must be compared with those obtained in children who are growing normally. Unfortunately, such comparisons are scant. Preliminary data from the studies of Spiliotis et al. (1), however, make the important point that most normal children have approximately eight pulses of growth hormone secretion every 24 hours. The children who are defined as growth-hormone-deficient by usual criteria may have reduced 24-hour growth hormone secretion or bursts of growth hormone that are similar to those in normal children. The correlation between physiological growth hormone secretion and the results of dynamic function tests for growth hormone reserve is far from satisfactory. Thus, children could be defined as growth-hormone-deficient by pharmacological testing and yet have apparently normal patterns of growth hormone release as shown by frequent sampling methods or, probably more commonly, can be considered to have impaired spontaneous growth hormone secretion with normal responses to dynamic function tests. It is not possible to delineate all of the factors that must be considered when evaluating such children, but obviously parental height, absence of disease, adequate nutrition, appropriate skeletal maturation, and lack of psychosocial problems should be considered. The interpretation of growth hormone values in the absence of such information is not rewarding.

A single basal Sm-C level is probably useful if it is normal. However, as mentioned above, nutritional factors play an important role in regulation of Sm-C secretion. Many of the Sm-C concentrations in mildly growth-retarded children are intermediate between those found in normal and hypopituitary children.

None of the tests of GH reserve have been standardized against responses in normal children. Most are standardized against responses of normal young adults, of siblings of growth-hormone-deficient children, or, even more curiously, in children with short stature who have "normal" responses. The most frequently used test is insulin-induced hypoglycemia. If performed under strict and well-supervised conditions, it is relatively benign. It may act by suppressing hypothalamic somatostatin secretion (17). The infusion of arginine has few side effects. The requirement for an infusion makes this somewhat more difficult to perform than some of the others. Arginine acts through the hypothalamus, although whether it acts to stimulate GHRH or to inhibit somatostatin or both is unknown. The oral administration of clonidine, an α_2-adrenergic agonist, may act by stimulating hypothalamic GHRH secretion (at least based on data in rats) (18). The disadvantage of the clonidine is that the time course of stimulation of GH is variable. Sampling, therefore, has to be continued for several hours. L-Dopa also has a variable time course of GH stimulation and is often associated with nausea. Its mechanism of action is unknown, but it almost certainly acts at the hypothalamic level to both stimulate GHRH and inhibit somatostatin secretion. Propranolol, the β-adrenergic blocking drug, cannot be used alone but may act by suppressing hypothalamic somatostatin release (19).

Growth hormone-releasing hormone can now be administered as an experimental drug. It was hoped that this agent would test GH reserve. However, there are several confounding factors. First, in normal adults GH responses to GHRH are extremely variable both among subjects and in the same subject on different occasions (20). This is almost certainly due to the fact that the response of the pituitary depends on the prevailing hypothalamic somatostatin secretion. Thus if GHRH is administered at a time when somatostatin secretion is low, there will be a large response. If GHRH is administered at a time when somatostatin levels are high, there will be a very small GH response.

Results of GHRH testing of children with short stature of varying etiologies can be summarized: 1.) Children with idiopathic short stature who do not meet the classic criteria for GH deficiency demonstrate an increase in GH in response to GHRH (see Figures 6 and 7). The responses are variable (20–23) as in normal young adults and in children at various stages of puberty. 2.) The same is true of most children with constitutional delay of growth and adolescence. 3.) Most children with idiopathic GH deficiency respond to GHRH, although in a few the responses are absent. 4.) Many children with organic hypopituitarism fail to respond to GHRH. This may result from the therapy that the

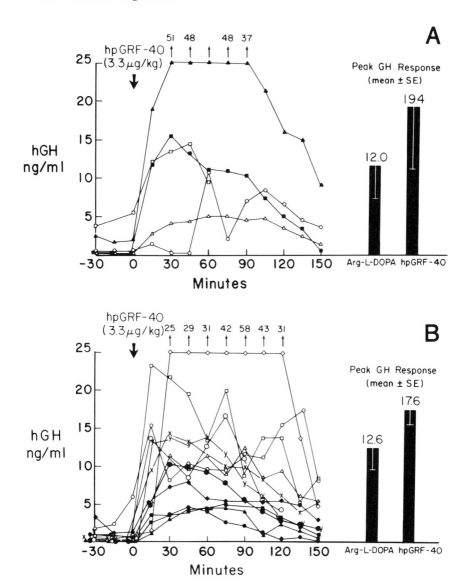

Figure 6. GH release in response to hGRF-40 in children with short stature. Each symbol represents an individual patient. (A) Intrauterine growth retardation and (B) constitutional delay of growth and adolescence and/or familial short stature. Bars at the right of each panel are the mean ±SEM of the peak GH responses to the arginine/L-dopa and hGRF-40. (From Ref. 22.)

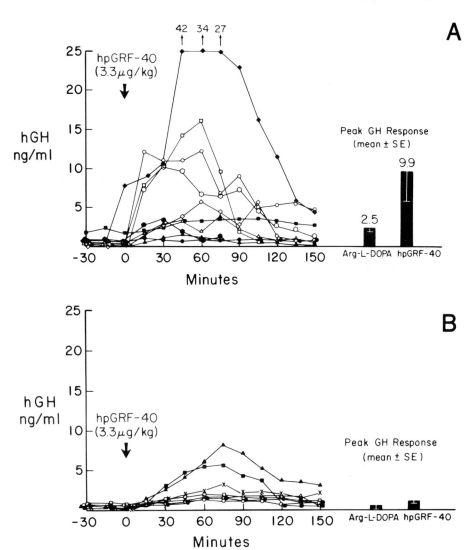

Figure 7. GH release in response to hGRF-40 in children with short stature. Each symbol represents an individual patient. (A) Isolated GH deficiency and (B) organic hypopituitarism. Bars at the right of each panel are the mean ±SEM of the peak GH responses to the arginine/L-dopa and hGRF-40. (From Ref. 22).

children have received rather than the disease process involving the pituitary.

If the GHRH test causes stimulation of GH secretion, it indicates that pituitary somatotropes are present and linked through GHRH receptors to allow GH secretion. Failure to respond could either be due to a defect at the level of the somatotrope or to the somatotrope not being previously exposed to GHRH. In the latter situation repeated injections of GHRH may be required to demonstrate that there is no pituitary defect. Failure to respond to GHRH could also result from excessive hypothalamic somatostatin secretion (Figures 6 and 7).

III. CONCLUSIONS

From this brief review it is clear that there are more questions than answers. We believe that more data on normal children are urgently required. The optimal frequency of sampling and the optimal duration of sampling need to be determined. At present the growth velocity of the child, the response to standard dynamic tests, and possibly the basal serum Sm-C concentration and/or the pattern of GH secretion over a 24-hour period appear to be the most useful. The GHRH test offers the opportunity of excluding a primary pituitary defect. Disturbances of GH secretion may result from neurosecretory disturbances that may be transient, or may represent part of the spectrum between normal variation and pathological GH secretion. Criteria to distinguish these possibilities are lacking at present.

REFERENCES

1. Spiliotis BE, August GP, Hung W, Sonis W, Mendelson W, Bercu BB. Growth hormone neurosecretory dysfunction: A treatable cause of short stature. J. Am. Med. Assoc. 152:2223–2251, 1984.

2. Ho KY, Evans WS, Blizzard RM, Veldhuis JD, Merriam GR, Samojlik E, Furlanetto R, Rogol AD, Kaiser DL, Thorner MO. Effects of sex and age on the 24 hour secretory profile of GH secretion in man: Importance of endogenous estradiol concentrations. J. Clin. Endocrinol. Metab. 64:51–58, 1987.

3. Gerich JE, Lorenzi M, Bier DM, Tsalikian E, Schneider V, Karam JH, Forsham PH. Effects of physiologic levels of glucagon and growth hormone on human carbohydrate and lipid metabolism: Studies involving administration of exogenous hormone during suppression of endogenous hormone secretion with somatostatin. J. Clin. Invest. 57:875, 1976.

4. Metcalfe P, Johnston DG, Nosadini R, Ørksov H, Alberti KGMM. Metabolic effects of acute and prolonged growth hormone excess in normal and insulin-deficient man. Diabetologia 20:123, 1981.

5. Sherwin RS, Schulman GA, Hendler R, Walesky M, Belous A, Tamborlane W. Effect of growth hormone on oral glucose tolerance and circulating metabolic fuels in man. Diabetologia 24:155, 1983.

6. Reichlin S. Neuroendocrinology. In Williams Textbook of Endocrinology, 7th ed., Wilson JD, Foster DW, eds., Saunders, Philadelphia, 1985, pp. 492–567.

7. Tannenbaum GS, Martin JB. Evidence for an endogenous ultradian rhythm governing growth hormone secretion in the rat. Endocrinology 98:562, 1976.

8. Ho KY, Furlanetto R, Alberti KGMM, Thorner MO. Fasting unmasks an intrinsic pulsatile pattern of GH secretion in man (abstract). The Endocrine Society, 68th Annual Meeting, Anaheim, Calif., 1986.

9. Soliman AT, Hassan AEHI, Aref MK, Hintz RL, Rosenfeld RG, Rogol AD. Serum insulin-like growth factors (IGF) I and II concentrations and growth hormone and insulin responses to arginine infusion in children with protein-energy malnutrition before and after nutritional rehabilitation. Pediatr. Res. 20:1122–1130, 1986.

10. Tannenbaum GS, Ling N. The interrelationship of growth hormone (GH)-releasing factor and somatostatin in generation of the ultradian rhythm of GH secretion. Endocrinology 115:1952, 1984.

11. Vance ML, Kaiser DL, Evans WS, Thorner MO, Furlanetto R, Rivier J, Vale W, Perisutti G, Frohman LA. Evidence for a limited growth hormone (GH)-releasing hormone (GHRH)-releasable quantity of GH: Effects of 6-hour infusions of GHRH on GH secretion in normal man. J. Clin. Endocrinol. Metabl. 60:370, 1985.

12. Vance ML, Evans WS, Thorner MO. Growth hormone secretion is augmented during 14 days of continuous growth hormone releasing

hormone infusion in normal man. Am. Fed. Clin. Res., 1986. (abstract).

13. Vance ML, Kaiser DL, Evans WS, Furlanetto R, Vale W, Rivier J, Thorner MO. Pulsatile growth hormone secretion in normal man during a continuous 24-hour infusion of human growth hormone releasing factor (1-40): Evidence for intermittent somatostatin secretion. J. Clin. Invest. 75:1584, 1985.

14. Chihara K, Kodana H, Kaji H, Kita T, Kashio Y, Okimura Y, Abe H, Fujika T. Augmentation by propranolol of growth hormone-releasing hormone-(1-44)-NH$_2$-induced growth hormone release in normal short and normal children. J. Clin. Endocrinol. Metab. 61:229, 1985.

15. Link K, Blizzard RM, Evans WS, Kaiser DL, Parker MW, Rogol AD. The effect of androgens on the pulsatile release and the twenty-four-hour mean concentration of growth hormone in peripubertal males. J. Clin. Endocrinol. Metab. 62:159, 1986.

16. Clark RG, Jansson JO, Isaksson O, Robinson ICAF. Intravenous growth hormone: Growth responses to patterned infusions in hypophysectomized rats. J. Endocrinol. 104:53, 1985.

17. Vance ML, Kaiser DL, Rivier J, Vale W, Thorner MO. Dual effects of GHRH infusion in normal men: Somatotroph desensitization and increase in releasable growth hormone. J. Clin. Endocrinol. Metab. 62: 591, 1986.

18. Miki N, Ono M, Schizume K. Evidence that opiatergic and alpha-adrenergic mechanisms stimulate rat growth hormone release via growth hormone releasing-factor (GRF). Endocrinology 114:1950, 1984.

19. Mauras N. Blizzard RM, Thorner MO, Rogol AR. Selective beta 1 adrenergic receptor blockade with atenolol enhances growth hormone releasing hormone-mediated growth hormone release in man. Metabolism 36:369–372, 1987.

20. Thorner MO, Rivier J, Spiess J, Borges JLC, Vance ML, Bloom SR, Rogol AD, Cronin MJ, Kaiser DL, Evans WS, Webster JD, MacLeod RM, Vale W. Human pancreatic growth-hormone-releasing factor selectively stimulates growth-hormone secretion in man. Lancet 1:24, 1983.

21. Vance ML, Borges JLC, Kaiser DL, Evans WS, Furlanetto R, Thominet JL, Frohman LA, Rogol AD, MacLeod RM, Bloom S, Rivier J,

Vale W, Thorner MO. Human pancreatic tumor growth hormone releasing factor (hpGRF-40): Dose response relationships in normal man. J. Clin. Endocrinol. Metab. 58:838, 1984.

22. Gelato M, Malozowski S, Caruso-Nicoletti M, Ross JL, Pescovitz OH, Rose S, Loriaux DL, Cassorla F, Merriam G. Growth hormone (GH) responses to GH-releasing hormone during pubertal development in normal boys and girls: Comparison to idiopathic short stature and GH deficiency. J. Clin. Endocrinol. Metab. 63:174, 1986.

23. Rogol AD, Blizzard RM, Johanson AJ, Furlanetto R, Evans WS, Rivier J, Vale W, Thorner MO. Growth hormone release in response to human pancreatic tumor growth hormone releasing factor-40 in children with short stature. J. Clin. Endocrinol. Metab. 59:580, 1984.

24. Thorner MO, Vance ML, Evans WS, Blizzard RM, Rogol AD, Ho K, Leong DA, Borges JLC, Cronin MJ, MacLeod RM, Kovaks K, Asa S, Horvath E, Frohman L, Furlanetto R, Klingensmith GJ, Brook C, Smith P, Reichlin S, Rivier J, Vale W. Physiological and clinical studies of GRF and GH. Rec. Prog. Horm. Res. 42:589, 1986.

6

Predictors of Response to Treatment with Methionyl Human Growth Hormone

BARRY M. SHERMAN, JAMES FRANE,
and ANN J. JOHANSON
Genentech, Inc.
South San Francisco, California

SELNA L. KAPLAN
University of California
at San Francisco
School of Medicine
San Francisco, California

Children with growth hormone deficiency have been treated with pituitary growth hormone for over 25 years. Nevertheless, the major predictors of response to treatment have not been clearly identified. Seventy-nine children with carefully documented GH deficiency have been followed during 1–4 years of treatment with Protropin, 0.1 mg/kg, (0.2 U/kg) intramuscularly three times weekly. The mean growth rate was greatest in the first year, 9.9 ± 2.4 cm/year, and was 6.5 ± 1.6 cm/year in year 4 in the 17 patients treated for 4 years. There was no correlation of the growth response and the pretreatment growth rate.

However, the first-year growth rate was highly correlated with that in later years. Patients with idiopathic GH deficiency ($n = 61$) had a first-year growth rate of 10.5 ± 2.4 cm/year, which was greater than that of 18 patients with organic etiologies, 8.4 ± 1.9 cm/year, $p = .002$. Patients with organic etiologies also had significantly greater mean height, weight, height age, and bone age. We used a variant of stepwise regression to explore the influence of 14 potential predictors of the growth response in patients with idiopathic GH deficiency. A model that accounted for 48% of the variability in the 12-month rate showed that a favorable response was best predicted by a lower basal somatomedin C concentration, a lower height age, greater adiposity, and greater maternal height. Since the growth rate in the first year of treatment is highly correlated with that in subsequent years, these predictors likely influence the overall response to GH therapy.

I. BACKGROUND

The treatment of GH deficiency using extracts from the human pituitary gland began in 1958 (1). Over the ensuing years, the supplies of pituitary hGH were limited and treatment was often interrupted. This interfered with effective assessment of long-term responses to GH treatment. Frasier reviewed many of the issues that surround the treatment of GH deficiency with pituitary GH (2).

Clinical studies of methionyl hGH produced by recombinant DNA technology began in 1981, and the subjects have now been carefully followed for as long as four years. This provides an opportunity to examine the long-term response to uninterrupted therapy and to assess some of the factors that influence and predict the growth response.

II. PATIENTS AND METHODS

Between 1981 and 1985, 79 children with documented GH deficiency were entered into five separate clinical trials at 17 medical centers. Sixty-one had idiopathic GH deficiency and 18 had organic causes. None had been treated with GH. Other pretreatment characteristics are shown in Table 1. Growth hormone deficiency was defined as a serum

Table 1. Baseline Characteristics of Subjects Treated with Methionyl Human Growth Hormone for Up to Four Years

Duration of treatment	Age (years)	% Male	Height (cm)	Weight (kg)	Height age (years)	Bone age (years)	Prestudy growth rate (cm/year)
1 year ($n = 33$)							
Mean	7.5	72.7	106.7	20.0	4.8	5.3	4.0
Standard deviation	3.2		17.7	9.9	2.7	2.9	1.3
2 years ($n = 12$)							
Mean	9.0	66.7	114.2	24.3	6.0	6.9	3.1
Standard deviation	3.4		16.5	9.2	2.6	3.3	1.2
3 years ($n = 17$)							
Mean	7.8	47.1	103.8	19.1	4.4	5.1	3.6
Standard deviation	3.4		17.0	8.4	2.5	2.7	0.8
4 years ($n = 17$)							
Mean	8.1	58.8	107.4	19.4	4.9	5.6	3.2
Standard deviation	3.1		15.1	6.9	2.3	2.6	1.1
Total ($n = 79$)							
Mean	7.0	63.3	107.4	20.3	5.0	5.6	3.6
Standard deviation	3.2		16.8	8.9	2.6	2.9	1.2

GH response of 7 ng/ml or less to at least two standard provocative tests of GH secretory capacity. All patients were treated with methionyl hGH at a dose of 0.1 mg/kg administered intramuscularly three times weekly. The dose was adjusted annually based on body weight. The growth response was assessed at 2-month intervals by trained observers using wall-mounted measuring devices. An x-ray of the left hand and wrist was taken every 6 months for assessment of bone age. Bone age was determined by a trained observer at the Fels Institute, Yellow Springs, Ohio. The somatomedin C concentration in samples from the first 46 subjects was measured by Dr. R. Hintz (3,4). The remainder were measured by radioimmunoassay at Genentech, Inc., using reagents supplied by Nichols Institute. Statistical methods included Student's *t*-test, Fisher's exact test, and all possible subsets regression, a variant of stepwise regression (5). Adiposity is expressed as the Quetelet index (1000 × weight/height; 2,6).

III. RESULTS

Table 2 shows the mean growth rate for children followed from 1 to 4 years. The average growth rate was 9.9 cm/year in the first year, 7.4 in the second, 7.1 in the third year, and 6.5 in the fourth year; it was unrelated to the pretreatment growth rate (Table 3). That is, there was no correlation between pretreatment and on-treatment growth rates in any year. By contrast, the growth rates in the first through third years of treatment were highly correlated, indicating that characteristic response patterns are sustained.

Prior to treatment, patients had bone age retardation ranging from 0.2 to 7.7, mean = 2.4 years. Table 4 shows that long-term GH therapy resulted in bone maturation that was synchronous with the increase in height with no evidence for accelerated bone maturation.

The dose of GH was adjusted annually, resulting in a year-to-year increase in the mean dose that reflected the increase in body weight (Table 4). The mean Sm-C concentration increased about threefold from baseline during the first year of treatment and continued to rise in the second and third years (Table 4).

Of the 79 subjects, 61 had idiopathic GH deficiency and had a first-year growth rate that was significantly greater than the 18 children

Table 2. Growth Rates (cm/year) for Each Year of Treatment

Duration of treatment	Age	Baseline	6 Months	First year	Second year	Third year	Fourth year
1 year (*n* = 33)							
Mean	7.5	4.0	10.5	9.5			
Standard deviation	3.2	1.3	3.3	2.6			
2 years (*n* = 12)							
Mean	9.0	3.1	10.7	9.6	7.9		
Standard deviation	3.4	1.2	2.9	2.5	2.1		
3 years (*n* = 17)							
Mean	7.8	3.6	12.3	10.4	7.5	7.2	
Standard deviation	3.4	0.8	2.1	2.2	1.9	1.9	
4 years (*n* = 17)							
Mean	8.1	3.2	10.4	10.4	7.0	7.0	6.5
Standard deviation	3.1	1.1	2.9	2.4	2.0	1.7	1.6
Total							
Mean	7.9	3.6	10.9	9.9	7.4	7.1	6.5
Standard deviation	3.2	1.2	3.0	2.4	2.0	1.8	1.6
n	79	79	79	79	46	34	17

Table 3. Correlations of Growth Rates during Three Years of Methionyl Human Growth Hormone Treatment

	Year 1	Year 2	Year 3
Prestudy	0.0586	0.1730	0.0500
Year 1		0.7232[a]	0.5961[a]
Year 2			0.7065[a]

[a]$p < .001$.

Table 4. Change in Height Age-to-Bone Age Ratio and Somatomedin C

	Baseline	First year	Second year	Third year	Fourth year
Delta HA/Delta BA					
n	—	77	44	24	—
Mean	—	1.5	1.2	1.1	—
Standard deviation	—	0.7	0.4	0.5	—
Somatomedin C (U/ml)					
n	77	79	46	34	17
Mean	0.3	0.9	1.3	1.7	1.8
Standard deviation	0.3	0.8	0.7	0.9	1.3

Delta bone age and delta height age are computed relative to baseline.

whose GH deficiency had organic causes, 10.4 ± 2.4 vs. 8.4 ± 1.9 cm/year, $p = .003$ (Table 5). The two groups did not differ significantly in age, sex distribution, basal Sm-C concentration, or parental height (Table 5). However, there were significant differences in several factors that might explain the difference in treatment response. The mean height, weight, height age, and bone age of patients with organic etiologies were significantly greater than in subjects with idiopathic GH deficiency (Table 5). Also, a greater proportion of patients with organic etiologies received glucocorticoid treatment, 8/18 vs. 6/61, $p = .002$.

We next used a variant of stepwise regression (all possible subsets regression) to explore possible predictors of the first-year growth response in patients with idiopathic GH deficiency. We examined the relationship between the 12-month growth rate and the following potential baseline predictor variables: sex, age, height, weight, height age, bone age, prestudy growth rate, father's height, mother's height, pretreatment Sm-C concentration, GH antibody status, thyroid hormone therapy, glucocorticoid therapy, maximal serum GH response during provocative testing, and the Quetelet index.

A model that included height age, basal Sm-C concentration, Quetelet index, and maternal height accounted for 48% of the variance in the first-year growth rate (Table 6).

Table 5. Baseline Characteristics of Subjects Treated with Methionyl Human Growth Hormone: Idiopathic versus Organic

	Age (years)	% Male	Height (cm)	Weight (kg)	Height age (years)	Bone age (years)	Prestudy growth rate (cm/yr)	Growth rate year 1 (cm/yr)	Somatomedin C (U/ml)
Idiopathic									
n	61	61	61	61	61	61	61	61	61
Mean	7.6	67.2	103.7	18.7	4.4	5.1	3.8	10.4	0.3
Standard deviation	3.2		15.2	7.5	2.3	2.7	1.2	2.4	0.3
Organic									
n	18	18	18	18	18	18	18	17	16
Mean	8.8	50.0	118.5	25.5	6.8	7.0	3.0	8.4	0.4
Standard deviation	3.2		17.7	11.3	2.8	3.0	1.2	1.9	0.3
Between-group comparisons									
t-statistic	1.39	—	3.51	3.11[a]	3.70	2.53	−2.41	−3.10	−0.02[a]
p value	0.167	0.266[b]	0.001	0.003	<0.001	0.013	0.018	0.003	0.982

[a]Based on log scale.
[b]Fisher exact test.

Table 6. Regression Equation for Estimating Growth Rate in First Year of Treatment of Patients with Idiopathic Growth Hormone Deficiency

	Regression coefficient	Standard error	t statistic	p value
Height age	−0.342	0.117	−2.92	.005
log(Sm-C)	−3.7	0.802	−4.61	<.0005
log(Quetelet index)	13.5	4.0	3.36	.001
Mother's height	0.093	0.033	2.81	.007
Intercept	−8.29			
Root mean squared error		1.82		
Squared multiple correlations		0.48		
F statistic		13.01		
Numerator degrees of freedom		4		
Denominator degrees of freedom		56		
Significance (tail probability)		<.00005		

$$
\begin{aligned}
\text{First-year growth response} = \ & - \ 8.29 \\
& - \ 0.342 \times \text{height age} \\
& - \ 3.70 \times \log 10 \ (\text{baseline Sm-C}) \\
& + 13.5 \times \log 10 \ (\text{Quetelet index}) \\
& + \ 0.0930 \times \text{mother's height}
\end{aligned}
$$

In other words, a better growth rate was predicted in patients who had a lower height age, a lower basal Sm-C concentration, greater adiposity, and taller mothers.

The mean pretreatment Quetelet index was 1.68 ± 0.26 at baseline and did not change during the first year of treatment, although there was a slight but statistically significant increase in the second through fourth years. The standard deviation of the yearly difference from baseline in the Quetelet index was less than 0.20, indicating little change in adiposity of individual subjects, as measured by this index.

IV. DISCUSSION

Human growth hormone produced by recombinant DNA methods is physiologically indistinguishable from material extracted from the human pituitary gland (7–9), and the initial responses of GH-deficient children to treatment with recombinant hGH are equivalent to results using pituitary hGH at the same dose (10). Previous studies of the responses of GH-deficient children to long-term treatment with pituitary GH were often compromised by limited supplies of the hormone and interruptions of therapy. The advantages of this study are related to the consistent treatment of a large, well-defined, carefully monitored group of GH-deficient children for up to 4 years. All children were treated with a dose of 0.1 mg/kg of Protropin three times a week, adjusted annually, a dose that is approximately twice that of pituitary GH traditionally employed.

The growth response was greatest in the first year and decreased somewhat thereafter, consistent with other studies reviewed by Frasier (2). Overall, 82% of the children in this study are growing at a rate of 6 cm/year or more. Seventy percent of children in the fourth year of treatment are growing more than 6.0 cm/year. As expected, plasma Sm-C concentrations increased after the initiation of GH treatment and were sustained at the same or higher levels for up to 4 years.

Despite many studies, there has been a lingering concern that GH treatment might accelerate bone maturation, leading ultimately to a reduction in growth potential. Accelerated bone maturation has not been observed in other studies employing pituitary GH (2) or in this study where methionyl hGH was used. In patients treated for as long as 4 years, the average ratio of the change in height age to change in bone age remained essentially equal to one.

It is important to recognize that when the dose is adjusted for increasing weight there is a high correlation of the growth rate in the first year with the growth response in ensuing years. Since the growth response patterns of individual subjects are maintained over several years, an understanding of the factors that influence the growth response is essential for optimal therapy.

When the 79 subjects were categorized according to etiologies, those with idiopathic GH deficiency had a significantly better growth response than those with organic causes, as noted by Milner et al. (11). Idiopathic GH deficiency is usually a lifelong disturbance, whereas GH deficiency due to a craniopharyngioma, other central nervous system tumor, or trauma usually occurs after a period of normal growth. Thus it is not surprising that subjects with organic causes had bone ages and height ages more appropriate for their chronological age (Table 5). This suggests that the more mature the individual subject at the time treatment is initiated, the less with be the growth response. In addition, subjects with organic causes were more frequently treated with glucocorticoids.

We examined alleged predictors of growth in the children with idiopathic GH deficiency using a variant of stepwise regression analysis (11–17). It was possible to identify several factors which together accounted for about 48% of the variability in the first-year growth response. Since the year-to-year growth rates are highly correlated, these predictors likely influence the long-term response to hGH. These could be classified as genetic, nutritional, and maturational influences and included the pretreatment Sm-C concentration, height age, the Quetelet index (a reflection of adiposity), and maternal height.

A better growth response was related to a lower baseline Sm-C concentration and lower height age, both of which might reflect the degree of GH deficiency. That is, less GH secretion results in a lower basal Sm-C concentration, greater growth retardation, and a less mature individual. Previous studies of GH-deficient children have not consistently shown this inverse relationship between basal circulating Sm-C concentration and the growth and metabolic responses to GH administration (18–20). The correlation observed in this study is probably related to the larger number of patients and the fact that none of them had previous treatment with GH.

There was no relationship between the posttreatment Sm-C concentration and the growth response, consistent with previous studies (18). Tables 2 and 4 show a decrease in mean growth rate after the first year of treatment and a simultaneous increase in the mean Sm-C concentration. The regulation of Sm-C in these circumstances is complex. The year-to-year increase in the mean Sm-C concentration could be related to the increase in absolute GH dose, but the subjects are also increasing in age, and age has been associated with a greater Sm-C response to GH administration (18). Changes in the sex hormone mi-lieu, as well as changes in the concentration of Sm-C binding protein, may also affect the circulating Sm-C concentration. At this time there is no adequate explanation for the diminution in growth rate in the face of an increasing Sm-C concentration.

Clinically, GH-deficient children have excess adipose tissue that seems to regress after initiation of treatment. Some physicians believe that a nutritional supplement improves an individual patient's growth response. These observations have led some to suggest that nutritional status might influence the growth response. The current study shows that a greater Quetelet index contributed favorably to the growth re-sponse. The Quetelet index was highly correlated with absolute weight ($r = .65$) and there was little individual variability in the Quetelet index over 2–4 years, suggesting that individual subjects maintained their relative degree of adiposity. Thus although a relatively poor nutritional status might impair the growth response, a decrease in adiposity is not likely to account for the diminished growth rate after the first year of treatment.

The other factor contributing to the initial growth response was a positive association with maternal height, undoubtedly reflecting the genetic contribution to growth potential. Since parental height was reported to the investigators rather than measured, the association of growth rate with maternal rather than paternal stature or both may reflect more accurate reporting of maternal height.

None of the factors examined is individually a strong predictor of the growth response, although together they account for nearly half of the variability in the first-year growth rate. Knowledge that patients who respond less well are those with organic etiologies, those who are thin, and those who have a greater height age or short parents may help to individualize the treatment of GH deficiency. Moreover, children who initially respond well continue to do so, and those who respond poorly are unlikely to improve their growth rate in the absence of some change in treatment strategy. Since a growth rate of about 6–7 cm/year is necessary for catch-up growth, children who are receiving GH re-placement therapy and who have growth rates less than 6 cm/ year should be reevaluated to assure compliance with the prescribed pro-gram and with an adequate diet. Until studies of optimal dose and treatment schedule are completed, empirical trials of daily GH administration or judicious increases in dose may be warranted in poor responders in order that they might achieve optimal growth rates and a near normal height.

ACKNOWLEDGMENT

We are grateful to the following investigators who participated in this study: Gilbert P. August, Jennifer J. Bell, Dennis Bier, Sandra L. Blethen, Robert Blizzard, David R. Brown, Thomas P. Foley, Jr., Joseph M. Gertner, Raymond L. Hintz, Nancy J. Hopwood, Rebecca T. Kirkland, Stephen LaFranchi, Leslie P. Plotnick, Ron Rosenfeld, Steven Seelig, Louis E. Underwood, and David T. Wyatt; to Douglas Frasier for helpful discussion; to Joyce Kuntze and Catherine Stoppani for clinical monitoring; and to Judy Zivick for secretarial support.

REFERENCES

1. Raben MS. Treatment of a pituitary dwarf with human growth hormone. J. Clin. Endocrinol. 18:901, 1958.

2. Frasier SD. Human pituitary growth hormone (hGH) therapy in growth hormone deficiency. Endocr. Rev. 4:155, 1983.

3. Furlanetto RW, Underwood LE, Van Wyk JJ, D'Ercole AJ. Estimation of somatomedin-C levels in normals and patients with pituitary disease by radioimmunoassay. J. Clin. Invest. 60:648, 1977.

4. Hintz RL, Liu F, Marshall LB, Chung D. Interaction of somatomedin-C with an antibody directed against the synthetic C-peptide region of insulin-like growth factor I. J. Clin. Endocrinol. Metab. 50:405, 1980.

5. Dixon WJ, Brown MB, Engleman L, Frane JW, Hill MA, Jennrich RI, Toporek JD. BMDP Statistical Software. Berkeley: University of California Press, 1983.

6. Keys A, Fidanza F, Karvonen MJ. Indices of relative weight and obesity. J. Chron. Dis. 25:329.

7. Rosenfeld RG, Aggarwal BB, Hintz RL, Dollar LA. Recombinant DNA-

derived methionyl human growth hormone is similar in membrane binding properties to human pituitary growth hormone. Biochem. Biophys. Res. Commun. 106:202, 1982.

8. Hintz RL, Rosenfeld RG, Wilson DM, Bennett A, Finno J, McClellan B, Swift R. Biosynthetic methionyl human growth hormone is biologically active in adult man. Lancet 1:1276, 1982.

9. Rosenfeld RG, Wilson DM, Dollar LA, Bennett A, Hintz RL. Both human pituitary growth hormone and recombinant DNA-derived human growth hormone cause insulin resistance at a postreceptor state. J. Clin. Endocrin. Metab. 54:1033, 1982.

10. Kaplan SL, August GP, Blethen SL, Brown DR, Hintz RL, Johanson AJ, Plotnick LP, Underwood LE, Bell JJ, Blizzard RM, Foley TP, Hopwood NJ, Kirkland RT, Rosenfeld RG, Van Wyk JJ. Clinical studies with recombinant DNA-derived methionyl human growth hormone in growth hormone deficient children. Lancet 1:697, 1986.

11. Milner RDG, Russell-Fraser T, Brook CGD, Cotes PM, Farquhar JW, Parkin JM, Preece MA, Snodgrass GJAI, Mason AS, Tanner JM, Vince FP. Experience with human growth hormone in Great Britain: The report of the MRC working party. Clin. Endocrinol. 11:15, 1979.

12. Tanner JM, Whitehouse RH, Hughes PCR, Vince FP. Effect of human growth hormone treatment for 1 to 7 years on growth of 100 children, with growth hormone deficiency, low birthweight, inherited smallness, Turner's syndrome and other complaints. Arch. Dis. Child. 46:745, 1971.

13. Preece MA, Tanner JM, Whitehouse RH, Cameron N. Dose dependence of growth response to human growth hormone in growth hormone deficiency. J. Clin. Endocrinol. Metab. 42:477, 1976.

14. Aceto T, Frasier SD, Hayles AB, Meyer-Bahlburg HFL, Parker ML, Munschauer R, DiChiro G. Collaborative study of the effects of human growth hormone in growth hormone deficiency. I. First year of therapy. J. Clin. Endocrinol. Metab. 35:483, 1972.

15. Aceto T, Frasier SD, Hayles AB, Meyer-Bahlburg HFL, Parker ML, Munschauer R, DiChiro G. Collaborative study of the effects of human growth hormone in growth hormone deficiency. III. First eighteen months of therapy. In Advances in Human Growth Hormone Research; A Symposium, U.S. Department of Health, Education and Welfare, Publication No. NIH 74-612, 1973, p. 695.

16. Guyda H, Friesen H, Bailey JD, Leboeuf G, Beck JC. Medical Research Council of Canada therapeutic trial of human growth hormone: First 5 years of therapy. Can. Med. Assoc. J. 112:1301, 1975.

17. Ranke M, Weber B, Bierich JR. Long-term response to human growth hormone in 36 children with idiopathic growth hormone deficiency. Eur. J. Pediatr. 132:221, 1979.

18. Rosenfeld RG, Kemp SF, Hintz RL. Constancy of somatomedin response to growth hormone treatment of hypopituitary dwarfism, and lack of correlation with growth rate. J. Clin. Endocrinol. Metab. 53: 611, 1981.

19. Schimpff RM, Donnadieu M, Gourmelen M, Girard F. The effects of hGH treatment of somatomedin levels in the serum. Horm. Metab. Res. 6:494, 1974.

20. Kastrup KW, Anderson H, Eskildsen PC, Jacobsen BB, Krabbe S, Petersen KE. Combined test of hypothalamic-pituitary function in growth retarded children treated with growth hormone. I. Secretion of growth hormone and somatomedin before and after treatment. Acta Paediatr. Scand. (Suppl.) 277:9, 1980.

7

Controversies in the Treatment of Short Stature

LOUIS E. UNDERWOOD
University of North Carolina
School of Medicine
Chapel Hill, North Carolina

BARRY M. SHERMAN
Genentech, Inc.
South San Francisco, California

INTRODUCTION

Over the past decade there has been growing awareness among pediatric endocrinologists that the capacity to define growth hormone deficiency is limited and not nearly as good as once thought. Whereas diagnosis is not difficult in children with severe unequivocal GH deficiency, uncertainty is common when the patient is able to secrete some GH. The source of the difficulties with diagnosis lies in the fact that there is no bimodal distribution of GH secretion by which the physician can distinguish short children who secrete insufficient hormone and would benefit from GH therapy from those who secrete adequate amounts of GH and do not need such therapy. In addition, the short-ages that preceded the advent of recombinant DNA-derived GH made it impossible to study adequately the relationship between GH secretion and responsiveness to therapy.

Most clinicians now agree that the discriminators of 7–9 ng/ml for peak serum GH responses to provocative stimuli are arbitrary and are not applicable universally. Additionally, doubt is growing about the closeness of the relationship between peak responsiveness to provocative stimuli and ability to secrete GH throughout the day. Because of this uncertainty, some investigators advocate the use of frequent or continuous sampling over many hours as a more reliable indicator of GH secretion. A significant shortcoming of such testing methods, however, is the lack of standardization with data from normal children and the near absence of data on the relationship between the amount of hormone detected by such testing methods and need for and response to therapy.

Deciding which short children should receive GH therapeutically is made even more difficult by recent observations by several groups of investigators whose studies suggest that children who appear not to be GH deficient will experience growth acceleration when treated. The accelerated growth of these so-called normal short or constitutional growth delay children raises questions about the value of exhaustive efforts to define a given patient's GH secretory status precisely. Other questions outstanding in such patients are whether their accelerated growth observed with months of therapy will last for years, whether their heights can be normalized, whether the gains made with treatment will persist when therapy is stopped, whether their adult heights will be changed by therapy, whether treatment will benefit them psychologically, and, finally, whether long-term treatment will produce late and unforeseen side effects.

To address these questions, a panel of experts on growth diagnosis and the therapeutic use of GH was assembled for this symposium. Rather than have each panelist discuss his or her area of expertise, we gathered from our files three cases of children with short stature, presented the panelists with their case histories and growth charts several weeks before the symposium, and asked them not only to comment on the cases but to address specific questions posed with each case. This format was chosen with the following objectives in mind:

1. To remove from the abstract panelists remarks concerning the diagnosis of GH deficiency and use of GH therapeutically, and to obtain opinions on specific patient-related issues.
2. To define in a practical context the points on which experts agree, and to expose and contrast the areas of uncertainty and disagreement.
3. To air in the context of actual cases some of the emotional and ethical problems that the physician must address before undertaking treatment of a short child with GH.

We believe that this effort at focusing the panelists' presentations was successful. As you study the pages that follow, note the uncertainty that is apparent in this area of inquiry, contrast the differences in opinion and approach among the experts, and know that you are not alone in your own uncertainty about the management of such patients.

CASE 1

This white boy was evaluated at 15.0 years of age because of short stature, delayed puberty, and adjustment difficulties. He was born normally after an uncomplicated 36-week gestation, and had a birth weight of 2.2 kg and length of 49 cm. At several days of age, he had an exchange transfusion because of jaundice, the result of ABO incompatibility. He also had a blood transfusion at 1 month because of anemia. He had no serious illnesses during infancy and childhood. He had a tonsillectomy at 2 years and infectious mononucleosis at 12 years. He was known to have been smaller than his peers for several years, but his size discrepancy had become more obvious 2–3 months earlier when the family moved to the United States from Latin America.

The family history is pertinent in that he has a 14-year-old brother whose height is below the 3rd percentile and who is sexually immature. Three younger siblings are of normal height. The boy's father, who is 172 cm (68 inches) tall and of Romanian and Mediterranean extraction, also experienced delayed puberty until he was 16 years old. The boy's mother is 158 cm (62 inches) tall.

On physical examination his height was 141.6 cm (height age, 11 years; Figure 1) and his weight was 32.3 kg (weight age, 10.7 years). He was well nourished and exhibited no physical abnormalities. The left testis measured 2.3 × 1.3 cm; the right testis measured 2.5 × 1.6

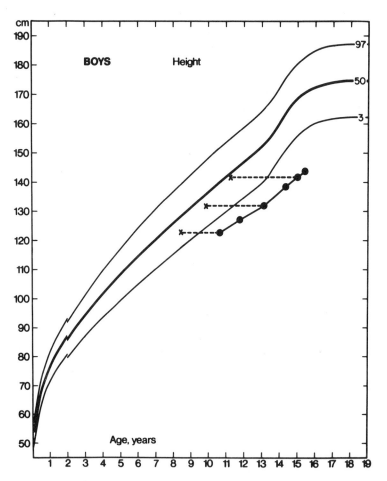

Figure 1.   Growth chart for the 15-year-old boy described in case 1.

cm. Pubic hair was Tanner Stage II, and there was thinning of the scrotal skin.

Serum testosterone was 31 ng/dl and plasma Sm-C/IGF-I was 1.4 U/ml. Skeletal age was 11 years. After the infusion of L-arginine, his maximal serum GH value was 11.4 ng/ml (60 minutes), and after insulin-induced hypoglycemia the maximal GH was 4 ng/ml. Assessment by a psychologist suggested that the patient was having psychological distress and appeared to be depressed. Psychotherapy was recommended.

At 15.3 years his height was 142.8 cm (growth rate, 3.5 cm/year). The left testis measured 2.4 × 1.3 cm, and the right testis measured 3.0 × 1.4 cm. No other changes in physical findings were noted.

Questions

1. Is this patient GH deficient? How do you interpret the results of the tests that were done?
2. What additional tests would you administer to determine whether he is GH deficient?
3. Would this patient benefit from GH therapy?
4. Are there methods for predicting whether he will have accelerated growth with GH therapy?
5. What treatment would you recommend for him?
6. Does this patient have ''bioinactive'' GH? Is there a means for testing for bioinactive GH?

Comments: Barry B. Bercu*

I believe that this young man has either a constitutional delay of growth and adolescence or a subtle deficiency in GH secretion. We know that he has been short for several years, but we know his growth pattern only since about 10.5 years of age. His stature was not a problem until the family moved to the United States. His present height puts him significantly below 2 SD (1). The normal Sm-C/IGF-I confuses the

---

*University of South Florida College of Medicine, St. Petersburg, Florida.

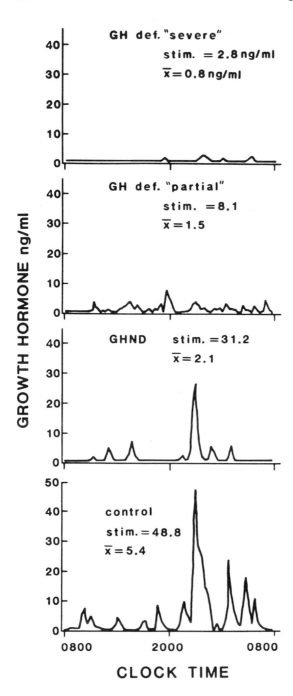

issue. It should be viewed as a screening procedure and placed in the context of the patient's total clinical and laboratory assessment. Provocative GH testing excludes "classical" GH deficiency, according to the criteria we have accepted for years. The information we are given about the psychological assessment does not allow us to discriminate between social and peer pressures stemming from his short stature, as opposed to environmental change. The latter could be important in this teenager, being precipitated by cultural differences resulting from moving to this country. Growth can be seasonal, so a 3-month period of observation is probably too short an interval to be certain of an annualized growth velocity. Nonetheless, taking the points from his growth chart over nearly 2 years, his growth velocity is approximately 5.3 cm/year, which is in the normal range. The recent onset of pubertal development and the minimal increase in testosterone are unlikely to have affected his growth velocity.

With regard to whether he is GH deficient, a 4-year delay in bone age is suggestive of but not definitive for an abnormality of GH secretion. The normal peak GH after L-arginine excludes classical GH deficiency based on a definition of blunted peak GH (arbitrarily less than 10 ng/ml in our laboratory). These results, however, do not eliminate GH deficiency as a result of decreased total output of GH and/or abnormal secretory pattern (2). We term such a disorder GH neurosecretory dysfunction (GHND), and we view it as a GH-deficient state. This point is further highlighted by the examples in Figures 2 and 3.

With regard to additional tests, I would like to do a 24-hour assessment of endogenous GH secretion. Traditional provocative test-

---

Figure 2. Representative example of the pulsatile GH secretion, stimulated peak GH after provocative testing (stim), mean ($\bar{x}$) 24-hour GH concentration in various groups of children. The arbitrary definitions used are based on peak GH response to two or more provocative tests (arginine, insulin, L-dopa, or clonidine) ("severe" GH deficiency = peak GH < 5 ng/ml, "moderate" GH deficiency = 5–7 ng/ml, "partial" GH deficiency = 7–9.9 ng/ml). GHND = GH neurosecretory dysfunction. Note that the total output of endogenous GH as expressed by 24-hour mean GH concentration may have no relationship to the peak GH value.

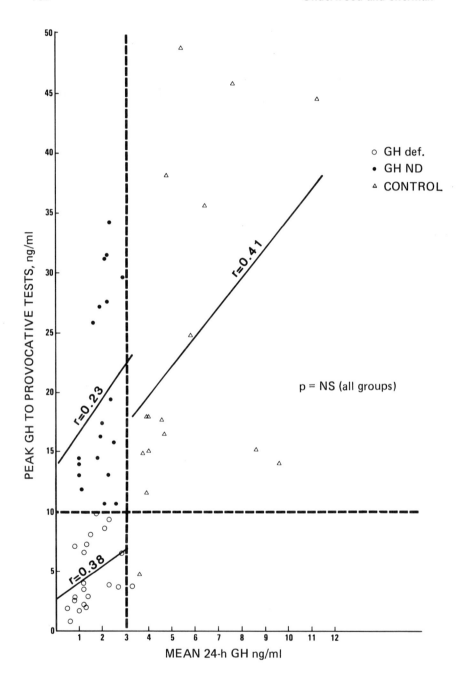

ing can be misleading when compared to endogenous secretion. We have recently shown that a 12-hour nocturnal study can give information similar to that of the complete 24-hour study.

I believe that the patient would probably benefit from GH therapy. Unfortunately, with this degree of bone age retardation it would be impossible to predict accurately his final height. The Greulich and Pyle charts are most useful only if his bone age of 11 is 1 year or less than his chronological age; obviously this is not the case. Then his predicted height would be 172 ± 5 cm but such a prediction is invalid. His parents' heights are 172 cm (father) and 158 cm (mother). If he had constitutional delay, without treatment one would expect him to reach a mature adult height between his parents' heights. I find it difficult to recommend a trial of exogenous GH therapy without having information on his 24-hour endogenous secretion of GH. However, I believe a 6-month trial of GH is appropriate for the following reasons:

1. His growth velocity of 3.5 cm/year in recent months is unsatisfactory. According to the Tanner growth velocity charts, only at a chronological age of 12.3 would such a growth velocity be within 2 SD.
2. A bone age delay of 4 years is unlikely to be caused only by constitutional delay of growth and adolescence. Unfortunately, such a diagnosis can only be made retrospectively.
3. His height puts him significantly below 2 SD of late maturers (1).
4. The goal would be to at least double his growth velocity over the next several months before he begins his pubertal growth spurt.

Figure 3. Correlation of mean 24-hour GH concentration to maximum peak GH concentration after provocative testing. The dashed line at 10 ng/ml peak GH represents the cutoff for normal peak GH concentration after provocative testing, and the dashed line at 3 ng/ml mean GH segregates normal and abnormal GH 24-hour mean concentration. Note the particularly poor correlations for the GH-deficient and GHND groups. In addition, the control group has significant variation.

Are there methods for predicting whether he will have accelerated growth with GH therapy? I think not. This patient already has an Sm-C/IGF-I in the normal range. He is in early puberty and the endogenous testosterone may be responsible for increasing the Sm-C/IGF-I concentration. The single low concentration of testosterone is still compatible with early puberty. Although early studies of the effect of short-term exogenous GH on Sm-C/IGF-I as a predictor for long-term therapeutic response were encouraging, more recent studies suggest that Sm-C/IGF-I generation is not predictive (3–5).

If he were treated, I would recommend at least 0.1 (0.05 mg) and preferably 0.2 U (0.1 mg) of GH per kilogram of body weight three times weekly for 6 months. A desirable increase in growth velocity would be to 7 cm/year or more, at least double his current growth velocity. An increase of at least 2 cm/year may be acceptable to some investigators, especially at the lower, more standard dose. In GH-deficient individuals an increase of another 30% in growth velocity with the higher dose would be expected (6,7).

Does this patient have "bioinactive" GH? At this point, there is no way to know whether this patient has a "bioinactive" GH molecule. Several methods have been used to search for such an entity. These have included measuring acute changes in plasma Sm-C/IGF-I after exogenous GH, and abnormal ratio of radioimmunoassay GH to radioreceptor assay (8–11). The IM-9 receptor modulation assay and the NB-2 lymphoma cell bioassay systems also have been utilized. A two-site immunoradiometric assay has also been used (12). I feel that none of these systems proves that the patient has "bioinactive" GH. What is necessary is proof of an abnormal amino acid sequence of the GH molecule.

References

1. Tanner JM, Davies PSW. Clinical longitudinal standards for height and weight velocity for North American children. J. Pediatr. 107:317–329, 1985.

2. Spiliotis B, August G, Hung W, Sonis W, Mendelson W, Bercu BB. Growth hormone neurosecretory dysfunction: A treatable cause of short stature. J. Am. Med. Assoc. 251:2223–2230, 1984.

3. Lanes R, Plotnick LP, Lee PA. Sustained effect of human growth

hormone therapy on children with intrauterine growth retardation. Pediatrics 63:731–735, 1979.

4. Rosenfeld RG, Kemp SF, Hintz RL. Constancy of somatomedin response to growth hormone treatment of hypopituitary dwarfism and lack of correlation with growth rate. J. Clin. Endocrinol. Metab. 53:611–617, 1981.

5. Van Vliet G, Styne DM, Kaplan SL, Grumbach MM. Growth hormone treatment for short stature. N. Eng. J. Med. 309:1016–1022, 1983.

6. Frasier SD. Human pituitary growth hormone (hGH) therapy in growth hormone deficiency. Endocr. Rev. 4:155–170, 1983.

7. Genentech, Inc. (unpublished data).

8. Kowarski AA, Schneider J, Ben-Galim E, Weldom VV, Daughaday WH. Growth failure with normal serum RIA-GH and low somatomedin activity: Somatomedin restoration and growth acceleration after exogenous GH. J. Clin. Endocrinol. Metab. 47:461–464, 1978.

9. Lanes P, Plotnick LP, Spencer ME, Daughaday WE, Kowarski AA. Dwarfism associated with normal serum growth hormone and increased bioassayable, receptorassayable, and immunoassayable somatomedin. J. Clin. Endocrinol. Metab. 50:485–488, 1980.

10. Rudman D, Kutner MH, Goldsmith MA, Kenney J, Jennings H, Bain RP. Further observations on four subgroups of normal variant short stature. J. Clin. Endocrinol. Metab. 51:1378–1384, 1980.

11. Tokuhiro E, Dean HJ, Friesen H, Rudman D. Comparative study of serum human growth measurements with N2 lymphoma cell bioassay, IM-9 receptor modulation assay and radioimmunoassay in children with disorders of growth. J. Clin. Endocrinol. Metab. 58:549–554, 1984.

12. Blethen SL, Chasalow FI. Use of a two-site immunoradiometric assay for growth hormone (GH) in identifying children with GH dependent growth failure. J. Clin. Endocrinol. Metab. 57:1031–1035, 1983.

Comments: S. Douglas Frasier*

If it is assumed that chronic underlying nonendocrine disease and hypothyroidism have been eliminated by appropriate studies in this

---

*University of California at Los Angeles School of Medicine, Los Angeles, and Olive View Medical Center, Sylmar, California.

patient, the remaining diagnostic considerations are 1.) severe constitutional delay in growth and adolescence; 2.) classical GH deficiency
and variants of GH deficiency such as nonclassical permanent GH
deficiency; 3.) transient GH deficiency, including that seen in psychosocial dwarfism and that which may accompany constitutional delay of
growth and adolescence (1,2).

The diagnosis of classical GH deficiency is not supported by at
least two pieces of laboratory information. The peak GH value after
the infusion of arginine of 11.4 ng/ml and the Sm-C/IGF-I value of
1.4 U/ml are outside of the range consistent with this diagnosis. However, this is a single GH test, and Sm-C/IGF-I is dependent on factors
other than GH. Therefore, these two pieces of information are not
conclusive. A history consistent with psychosocial dwarfism is not
present, and I do not think that this diagnosis needs to be given further
consideration.

I think that some additional studies of GH function should be
carried out. I would perform at least one other stimulation test using
either dopa or clonidine. A normal response to the additional stimulus
would further eliminate classical GH deficiency from consideration. If
the response to the additional stimulus was subnormal, I would repeat
testing with all three stimuli after androgen pretreatment in order to
focus on the differential between GH deficiency and constitutional
delay (3). I would interpret any equivocal or subnormal response prior
to androgen and a normal response after priming as supporting a diagnosis of constitutional delay. Others would argue that these results
were also consistent with some forms of nonclassical permanent GH
deficiency, such as neurosecretory dysfunction (4) or bioinactive GH.
Neurosecretory dysfunction might be studied by evaluating the 24-
hour pattern of GH secretion, although I believe interpretation of these
results remains unclear. The question of bioinactive GH can be studied
by determining GH activity by radioreceptor assay and comparing this
with a standard radioimmunoassay. Although bioinactive growth hormone exists (5), this method of study does not necessarily provide
uniformly interpretable results (6,7). Perhaps the use of monoclonal
antibodies in the immunoassay might better focus on this problem (8).

I believe that additional studies probably would support a diagnosis of severe constitutional delay of growth and adolescence with or

without associated transient GH deficiency. How might such a patient be treated? I do not believe that there are any methods available for predicting whether the patient would have accelerated growth in response to GH therapy. If the diagnostic studies supported severe constitutional delay without transient GH deficiency, in that androgen priming led to normal GH responsiveness, I probably would administer androgens as the treatment of choice (9,10). On the other hand, if transient GH deficiency accompanied severe constitutional delay and the patient had not responded after androgen priming, a trial of GH would be indicated and might result in significant acceleration of growth. Perhaps under these circumstances a combination of monthly testosterone injections and GH given in a standard fashion would be optimal. I believe that the initial dose of these agents should be no more than 100 mg of long-acting testosterone each month and no more than 0.1 IU of growth hormone per kilogram of body weight three times each week (11).

References

1. Trygstad O. Transitory growth hromone deficiency successfully treated with human growth hormone. Acta Endocrinol. 84:11–22, 1977.

2. Gourmelen M. Pham-Huu-Trung MT, Girard F. Transient partial hGH deficiency in prepubertal children with delay of growth. Pediatr. Res. 13:221–224, 1979.

3. Martin LG, Grossman MS, Connor TB, Levitsky LL, Clark JW, Camitta FD. Effect of androgenon growth hormone secretion and growth in boys with short stature. Acta Endocrinol. 91:201–212, 1979.

4. Spiliotis BE, August GP, Hung W, Sonis W, Mendelson W, Bercu BB. Growth hormone neurosecretory dysfunction. A treatable cause of short stature. J. Am. Med. Assoc. 251:2223–2230, 1984.

5. Valenta LJ, Sigel MB, Lesniak MA, Ellas AN, Lewis UJ, Friesen HG, Kershnar AK. Pituitary dwarfism in a patient with circulating abnormal growth hormone polymers. N. Engl. J. Med. 312:214–216, 1985.

6. LaFranchi S, Hanna CE, Jelen B. Growth hormone assessment by radioreceptor and radioimmunoassay. Am. J. Dis. Child. 138:23–27, 1984.

7. Tokuhiro E, Dean HJ, Friesen HG, Rudman D. Comparative study of

serum growth hormone measurement with NB2 lymphoma cell bio-assay, IM-9 receptor modulation assay, and radioimmunoassay in children with disorders of growth. J. Clin. Endocrinol. Metab. 58:549–554, 1984.

8. Blethen SL, Chasalow FI. Use of a two-site immunoradiometric assay for growth hormone (GH) in identifying children with GH-dependent growth failure. J. Clin. Endocrinol. Metab. 57:1031–1035, 1983.

9. De Lange WE, Snoep MC, Doorenbos H. The effect of short-term testosterone treatment in boys with delayed puberty. Acta Endocrinol. 91:177–183, 1979.

10. Rosenfeld RG, Northcraft GB, Hintz RL. A prospective, randomized study of testosterone treatment of constitutional delay of growth and development in male adolescents. Pediatrics 69:681–687, 1982.

11. Frasier SD. Human pituitary growth hormone (hGH) therapy in growth hormone deficiency. Endocrinol. Rev. 4:155–170, 1983.

Comments: Harvey J. Guyda*

This patient is *not* GH deficient. He has the typical features of a moderately severe delayed puberty or ''constitutional'' familial growth disturbance. I interpret his laboratory data as normal since it is not unusual to see variable GH responses, including poor responses, to provocative tests in otherwise normal children. The normal pubertal Sm-C/IGF-I concentration is strongly against GH deficiency of any type.

I would not recommend any additional GH tests since the boy already has psychic distress and is concerned about his normalcy. Additional tests would only support, in his mind, the idea that something is abnormal or that we are not sure of his diagnosis.

Having said this, I would have preferred a more physiological GH assessment such as a 6-hour daytime spontaneous secretion that we employ (1), nighttime secretion, or assessment of 24-hour mean GH secretion. It is likely that he has below average spontaneous GH secre-

*Montreal Children's Hospital and McGill University, Montreal, Quebec, Canada.

tion that would increase with either endogenous puberty or exogenous sex steroid administration. The term "transient" or "partial" GH secretion has been used by some researchers to describe this self-correcting phenomenon. (2).

I do not feel that his height would "benefit," in the long term, from GH therapy. However, he might benefit psychologically in the short term from either androgen or GH therapy for 6 months.

I do not believe that there are any methods available to predict growth responses to GH therapy. Giving him GH for 6–12 months *will* be associated with acceleration of his growth velocity since he is already in his pubertal growth spurt.

Given this, I would offer psychological support. If his psychological assessment indicates a need for active intervention, I would consider a short course (e.g., 3 months) of androgens after a careful explanation of his growth disorder and his normal height prognosis of 172 cm.

My negative opinion regarding the merit of GH therapy in boys with constitutional delay is based on personal experience and my interpretation of the literature. Ten years ago, we reported transient or partial GH deficiency in five patients with subnormal GH responses (<5 ng/ml) to ITT and ATT, but normal interval growth velocity and bone ages. Two of these patients did not benefit from 6 months of GH therapy (3). Figures 4 and 5 illustrate two additional recent cases treated with GH for 3–4 years with no real benefit, despite GH testing that suggested partial or sex steroid–dependent GH deficiency. Both patients asked to have GH discontinued and were very disappointed at the outcome.

The patient under discussion does not have "bioinactive" GH. There are no good tests available to determine if bioinactive GH is present, and I do not believe that a case of bioinactive GH has ever been documented. Assays using animal tissue receptors are imprecise and difficult to interpret. Furthermore, it is difficult to accept this diagnosis in any patient who achieves a normal growth rate for the first 5–10 years of life, or achieves normal adult height.

The patient reported by Valenta et al. (4) grew at a normal velocity for the first 10 years of his life, and had normal pubertal concentrations of Sm-C/IGF-I when first assessed, making the diagnosis

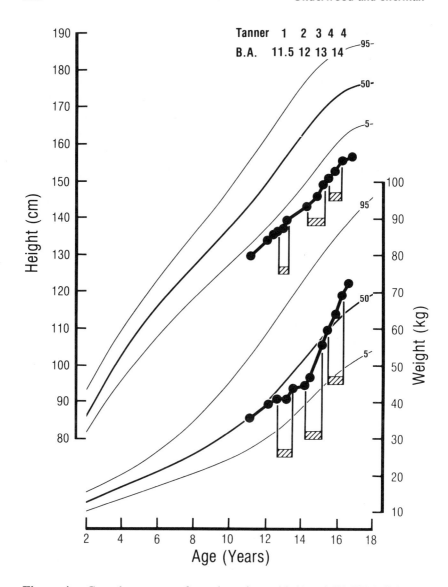

Figure 4. Growth response of a male patient with "partial" GH deficiency to 4 years of intermittent GH therapy (6 IU/week for 10/12 months). GH values were <5 ng/ml to ATT (2 ng/ml), ITT (3.5 ng/ml), and during a 6-h daytime GH profile (1.3 ng/ml). Bone age and puberty advanced during GH therapy without any obvious pubertal growth spurt. He was restudied following completion of puberty and had normal GH responses.

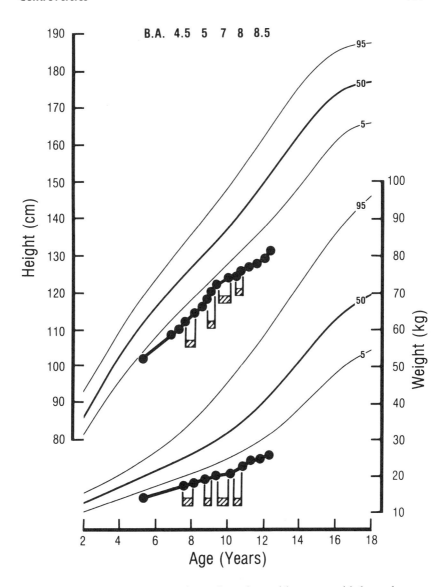

Figure 5. Growth response of a male patient with sex-steroid-dependent or "transitory" GH deficiency to four courses of GH treatment (6 IU/week). His peak spontaneous GH value after estrogen priming was 17.9 ng/ml. His bone age remained significantly delayed after 3 years of GH therapy and, on retesting 6 months after GH was stopped, he had GH values of 7.4 ng/ml (ATT), 3.3 ng/ml (ITT), and 3.6 ng/ml (6-h profile).

of a congenitally defective or "bioactive" GH molecule most unlikely. In addition, this patient had only a 25% decrease in bioactivity
as assessed by the NB2 rat lymphoma assay, but a 50% decrease in
receptor-reactive GH in the IM-9 cultured lymphocyte assay. Furthermore, when the original patients of Tokuhiro, Dean, Friesen, and
Rudman were reexamined in the NB2 and IM-9 assays, all values were
normal (5).

References

1. Miller JD, Tannenbaum GS, Colle E, Guyda HJ. Daytime pulsatile GH
   secretion during childhood and adolescence. J. Clin. Endocrinol. Metab.
   55:989–994, 1982.

2. Gourmelen M, Pham-Huu-Trung MT, Girard F. Transient partial hGH
   deficiency in prepubertal children with delay of growth. Pediatr. Res.
   13:221–224, 1979.

3. Tse WJ, Guyda HJ, Hoy P. Provocative tests for GH release. J. Pediatr.
   88:565–568, 1976.

4. Valenta LJ, Sigel MB, Lesniak MA, Ellas AN, Lewis UJ, Friesen HG,
   Kershnar AK. Pituitary dwarfism in a patient with circulating abnormal
   growth hormone polymers. N. Engl. J. Med. 312:214–216, 1985.

5. Tokuhiro E. Dean HJ, Friesen HG, Rudman D. Comparative study of
   serum human growth hormone measurement with NB2 lymphoma cell
   bioassay, IM-9 receptor modulation assay, and radioimmunoassay in
   children with disorders of growth. J. Clin. Endocrinol. Metab. 58:549–
   554, 1984.

6. Guyda H. Diagnosis and treatment of growth hormone deficiency. In
   Clinical Neuroendocrinology, Collu R, Brown GM, Van Loon GR, eds.,
   Blackwell Scientific, Boston, in press, 1987.

Editors' Note

This patient was treated with growth hormone (0.1 mg/kg three times
weekly) and testosterone (100 mg/month) for several months. His
growth rate increased dramatically, to 17 cm/year. More importantly,
he experienced an impressive improvement in his psychological status,
seeming to benefit greatly from this treatment.

CASE 2

This white boy was referred at 9.8 years for evaluation of short stature. He had been the product of an uncomplicated pregnancy and was delivered at term. His birth weight was 3100 g. His infancy was uneventful, but he was noted to have a length below the 3rd percentile at 18 months of age. He has been in excellent health throughout childhood, but his growth has remained slightly below the 3rd percentile. Recently, the boy was the subject of teasing by schoolmates and was manhandled on several occasions, which led to some overt psychological stresses.

At 4.7 years he was evaluated by the referring physician, who found him to have normal CBC, urinalysis, blood sugar, BUN, and thyroid function tests. His bone age was 3.5 years. His serum GH concentration rose to 21 ng/ml 60 minutes after ingesting L-dopa.

This boy's mother is 157 cm (62 inches tall) and his father is 170 cm (67 inches) tall. Paternal and maternal grandfathers are known to be 172.5 cm (68 inches) tall. No relatives are unusually short, and it is not known whether the father or other ancestors had delayed pubertal development. Two sisters are said to be of average height.

At 9.8 years his height was 123.6 cm (height age, 7.4 years; Figure 6) and his weight was 22 kg (weight age, 6.8 years). His vital signs and physical examination were completely normal. He had no pubertal development and his right testis measured 2.0 × 1.4 cm; left, 1.8 × 1.4 cm. His bone age was 7 years. His adult height from the tables of Bayley-Pinneau was predicted to be 172.5 cm (68 inches).

At 10.2 years his pituitary function was evaluated and revealed that his maximal GH after L-arginine infusion was 17.5 ng/ml, and after insulin-induced hypoglycemia it was 24.8 ng/ml. His serum GH peaked at 34.4 ng/ml 75 minutes after the onset of sleep. Basal TSH was 3.7 μU/ml, and TSH 30 minutes after injection of TRH was 12.5 μU/ml. Serum T_4 was 8.4 μg/dl, morning cortisol was 27.6 μg/dl, and plasma Sm-C/IGF-I was 1.3 U/ml.

At 10.25 years his height was 125.1 cm (growth rate, 3.9 cm/ year).

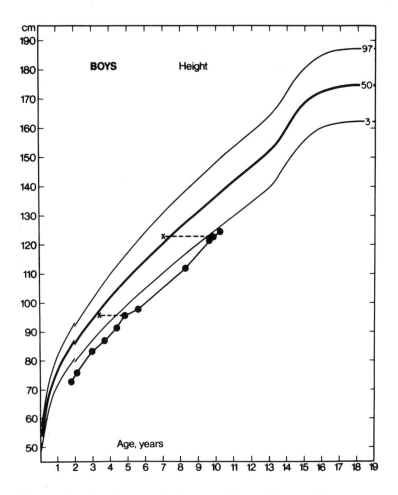

Figure 6. Growth chart for the boy discussed in case 2.

Questions

1. What is the patient's diagnosis?
2. Is GH rate-limiting for his growth?
3. What other tests might be helpful?
4. Should he be treated with GH?
5. If treated, what would be the response in terms of linear growth? What growth rate would you accept as indicative of a significant, worthwhile response to GH therapy?
6. What possible adverse side effects of GH therapy concern you in a patient like this?

Comments: John S. Parks*

The child in question has a growth pattern consistent with constitutional delay of growth and, by extrapolation, delay of pubertal development. His skeletal maturity is 2.8 years behind the standards of Greulich and Pyle and about 2 years behind the level appropriate for a more diverse and contemporary NCHS sample (1). Predicted mature height is an inch above the 25th percentile heights of his parents. The only unusual feature of his growth pattern is that he has grown at a steady rate of 6.0 cm/year between ages 5.5 and 9.8 years. This has brought him 4 cm closer to both the 3rd percentile of the Whitehouse and Tanner growth chart and the 5th percentile of the NCHS chart. The stated growth rate of 3.9 cm/year between 9.8 and 10.25 years reflects an inappropriately short sampling interval for prediction of future growth. Height for bone age has improved from the 25th to nearly the 75th percentile.

There is considerable evidence that diminished GH secretion does not account for this child's growth pattern. His peak GH values with arginine infusion, insulin-induced hypoglycemia, and sleep are well beyond the arbitrary levels of 7–10 ng/ml used as a criterion for diagnosis of classical GH deficiency. A single Sm-C/IGF-I value of 1.3 U/ml suggests that further attempts to link his short stature to diminished secretion or biological activity of GH would be fruitless.

Except in the context of a research protocol, I would not assess

---

*Emory University School of Medicine, Atlanta, Georgia.

24-hour patterns of GH secretion in this child. The child's pace of growth and his stimulted GH values are too normal for such a test to be of diagnostic value. Very little attention has been paid to the consistency of repetitive 24-hour sampling in the same child (2,3). It he did have an integrated GH concentration below 3 ng/ml, one might easily maintain that it was not representative of his ability to secrete GH and had little to do with his potential for responding to GH treatment. Comparison of radioreceptor to radioimmunoassay estimates of GH concentration (4–7) and attempts to disclose abnormal patterns of immunoreactivity with two or more monoclonal antibodies (8–10) would also have questionable diagnostic relevance. We have a research interest in the use of restriction fragment length polymorphism (RFLP) linkage analysis to determine the genetic basis of normal variation in the pace and extent of growth. Our hypothesis is that study of transmission of alleles for releasing and release-inhibiting peptides, GH, Sm-C/IGF-I, IGF-II, and hormone receptors will disclose major gene effects on growth. These studies are much too preliminary to use in a diagnostic context.

Reasonable screens for systemic illness were performed when the child was 4.7 years of age. His normal growth since that time and his weight for stature in the 25th percentile do not suggest either chronic disease or inadequate nutrition. Nevertheless, I would order a more inclusive chemistry screening panel, repeat a CBC, and order an erythrocyte sedimentation rate. I would not be inclined to order more specific tests for inflammatory bowel disease, gluten-sensitive enteropathy, or giardial infestation unless screening studies provided a potential lead. I would trust my physical examination to exclude or suggest microcephaly, disproportionate short stature, congenital heart disease, and chronic lung disease.

This child should not be treated with GH unless all parties understand and accept the experimental nature of such an undertaking. His shortness is a nuisance to him and his family. Viewed objectively, it is not severe enough to constitute a serious handicap. Instructions in prickliness and self-preservation and encouragement to learn sports that require skill rather than bulk would bring a better return than would an investment in biosynthetic GH.

There has been a great deal of debate about pretreatment predictors of GH response in short children without GH deficiency. Integrated growth hormone concentrations, pretreatment Sm-C/IGF-I concentration, and acute Sm-C/IGF-I responses to GH, low pretreatment height velocities, degree of shortness, and degree of bone age delay have all had their advocates and their debunkers (11–19). Conclusions depend on the doses of GH used and the duration of treatment. Most studies have used short-term outcome measures involving changes in height velocity over 6–12 month treatment periods. There has been insufficient attention to long-term effects.

In my opinion a growth rate which moved this child from below the 3rd to above the 10th percentile channel within 12 months is significant. This would require a growth rate of approximately 10 cm/year. However, I am not sure that such an exuberant growth rate would be worthwhile. Consider the long-term implications and objectives. We assume that we have achieved the short-term objective of moving the child to a significantly higher position in comparison to his age peers. Would GH need to be continued until maturity to keep him there? His pretreatment growth rate was normal. Would it decline to a subnormal value with interruption of treatment, reflecting a compensatory adjustment after an abnormal stimulus to growth? If GH were to be continued, would it be done with the objective of sustaining a height in the 10th percentile or with an objective of increasing adult height beyond the normal 68-inch height prediction? Our knowledge on this score is as primitive as the knowledge about the long-term effects of androgen treatment three decades ago. Until experience is gained on an experimental basis in large numbers of children followed from the start of treatment through completion of growth, we cannot address these questions as they apply to the individual child.

Our unpublished experience with long-term and necessarily intermittent GH treatment is pertinent to the general question of growth response. Dr. Robert Russell and I have followed the boys in Table 1. Eight boys were selected because of short stature and low Sm-C/IGF-I, and subsequently for a favorable initial growth response to GH therapy. Seven were started on treatment by Dr. Daniel Rudman in Atlanta and patient 1 was started by Dr. A. Kowarski in Baltimore (4). Doses were randomized between 0.15 and 0.75 U/kg/week. Mean pretreatment growth rate was 4.2 cm/year and all showed a 2.5 cm/

Table 1. Results of Long-Term GH Treatment

Growth Rates in Non-GHD Short Stature

Patient	First GH (cm/yr)	Later GH (cm/yr)	Off GH (cm/yr)	Dose depend
1	11.5	4.9	3.0	+
2	10.4	7.5	2.4	+
3	9.6	5.8	3.3	+
4	8.4	7.3	2.7	−
5	10.9	6.2	3.2	+
6	12.9	8.3	6.3	−
7	7.4	7.6	5.8	−
8	7.9	5.2	4.0	−
Mean	9.9	6.2	3.8	+/−

Net Effects of Long-Term Treatment

Patient	At start of GH			At last exam		
	CA	CA-BA	-SD	CA	CA-BA	-SD
1	3.8	1.8	4.6	11.0	3.0	3.3
2	3.5	1.5	3.6	6.8	1.8	2.8
3	7.9	2.9	3.1	12.1	3.6	2.8
4	6.9	0.9	2.2	11.8	0.3	1.6
5	7.1	2.6	3.0	13.1	1.1	2.5
6	9.5	5.0	5.0	12.0	6.0	3.5
7	7.0	2.5	2.5	12.1	2.1	1.3
8	8.2	2.7	3.8	11.2	3.7	3.6
Mean	6.7	2.5	3.5	11.3	2.7	2.7

year improvement during the first 6–12 months. In 7 of 8, growth rate during the first interval was greater than in any subsequent treatment interval. Half the children seemed to show a dependence on dose during the later periods. The net effect in five has been a maintenance of their pretreatment height percentiles. Aside from a nagging uncertainty about Creutzfeldt-Jakob disease, they are no better and no worse off than a typical untreated child with constitutional delay of growth. In fact, their mean growth rate on treatment after the first interval is no better than the child presented and discussed here experienced without treatment. Two of our patients (Table 1) have jumped from below the 5th to above the 10th percentile for height. We do not know what else distinguishes these two from the other children. We do not know, for example, whether administered GH supplemented rather than suppressed spontaneous GH secretion. One narrowed his bone age gap, entered puberty at an average age, and has continued rapid growth off treatment without a discernible effect on predicted mature height. His performance would not be unusual in a youngster treated with androgens from an early age. The experience with continuous higher dose biosynthetic GH may prove to be different, but we need to be very cautious about extrapolation to adult height from brief treatment experiences.

The short-term side effects that I worry about are largely psychological. One is the disappointment and frustration associated with failure to achieve a significant increase in growth. With the patient in question, the probability of an increase of more than 2.5 cm/year above his normal 6 cm/year pretreatment rate is probably less than 50%. The chances of a growth rate approximating 10 cm/year are even slimmer. If there is a minimal response, then this would be a heavy burden for a family that, by history, seems to regard their child as a loser. There is the more cerebral objection that treatments, especially powerful and expensive injection treatments, are given for a disease and that this child's slow but ultimately normal growth reflects a disease process. I am also concerned about the temptation to increase GH dose if the initial high dose does not produce success. We know that the GH excess of pituitary gigantism and acromegaly takes many years to produce kyphoscoliosis, myopathy, neuropathy, glucose intolerance, and premature death from hypertension and arteriosclerotic heart disease. We do not know the extent of GH excess needed to produce these side effects. Some young acromegalics produce 100 times the normal amount of GH, but in others a threefold or fourfold increase above normal production rates of 1–2 mg/day may be sufficient to produce morbidity.

References

1. Roche AF, Roberts J, Hamill PVV. National Center for Health Statistics: Skeletal maturity of children 6–11 years, United States. Vital and Health Statistics. Series 11-No. 140. DHEW Pub. No. (HRA) 75–1622. Health Resources Administration, Washington, U.S. Government Printing Office, 1975.

2. Spiliotis BE, August GP, Hung W, Sonis W, Mendelson W, Bercu BB. Growth hormone neurosecretory dysfunction. A treatable cause of short stature. J. Am. Med. Assoc. 251:2223–2230, 1984.

3. Thompson RG, Rodriguez A, Kowarski A. Integrated concentrations of growth hormone correlated with plasma testosterone and bone age in preadolescent and adolescent males. J. Clin. Endocrinol. Metab. 35:334–337, 1982.

4. Kowarski AA, Schneider J, Ben-Galim E, Weldon VV, Daughaday WH. Growth failure with normal serum RIA-GH and low somatomedin activity: Somatomedin restoration and growth acceleration after exogenous GH. J. Clin. Endocrinol. Metab. 47:461–464, 1978.

5. Rudman D, Kutner MH, Goldsmith MA, Kenny J, Jennings H, Bain RP. Further observations on four subgroups of normal variant short stature. J. Clin. Endocrinol. Metab. 51:1378–1383, 1980.

6. Frazer T, Gavin JR, Daughaday WH, Hillman RE, Weldon VV. Growth hormone-dependent growth failure. J. Pediatr. 101:12–15, 1982.

7. Tokuhiro E. Dean HJ, Friesen HG, Rudman D. Comparative study of serum human growth hormone measurement with NB2 lymphoma bioassay, IM-9 receptor modulation assay, and radioimmunoassay in children with disorders of growth. J. Clin. Endocrinol. Metab. 58:549–554, 1984.

8. Blethen S, Chasalow F. Use of a two-site immunoradiometric assay for growth hormone (GH) in identifying children with GH-dependent growth failure. J. Clin. Endocrinol. Metab. 57:1031–1035, 1983.

9. Blethen SL, Chasalow F, Bieser K. Immunologic heterogeneity of circulating hGH. Abstracts of the 7th International Congress of Endocrinology, Excerpta Medica International Congress Series 652. Abstract 115, 1984.

10. Agarwal S, Chalew S, Dhawan S, Kowarski A. Binding of GH to IM-9 cells involves the portion associated with its bioactivity. Abstracts of the 7th International Congress of Endocrinology, Excerpta Medica International Congress Series 652. Abstract 110, 1984.

11. Tanner JM, Whitehouse RH, Hughes PCR, Vince FP. Effect of human growth hormone treatment for 1 to 7 years on growth of 10 children, with growth hormone deficiency, low birthweight, inherited smallness, Turner's syndrome, and other complaints. Arch. Dis. Child. 46:745–782, 1971.

12. Grunt JA, Enriquez AR. Acute and long-term responsiveness to growth hormone in children with short stature. Pediatr. Res. 6:664–674, 1972.

13. Rudman D, Kutner MH, Blackston RD, Jansen RD, Patterson JH. Normal variant short stature: Subclassification based on responses to exogenous growth hormone. J. Clin. Endocrinol. Metab. 49:92–99, 1979.

14. Rudman D, Kutner MH, Blackston RD, Cushman RA, Bain RP, Patterson JH. Children with normal-variant short stature: Treatment with human growth hormone for six months. N. Engl. J. Med. 305:123–131, 1981.

15. Hayek A, Peake GT. Growth hormone and somatomedin-C responses to growth hormone in dwarfed children. J. Pediatr. 99:868–862, 1981.

16. Van Vliet G, Styne DM, Kaplan SL, Grumbach MM. Growth hormone treatment for short stature. N. Engl. J. Med. 309:1016–1022, 1983.

17. Plotnick LP, Van Meter QL, Kowarski AA. Human growth hormone treatment of children with growth failure and normal growth hormone levels by immunoassay: Lack of correlation with somatomedin generation. Pediatrics 71:324–327, 1983.

18. Bright GM, Rogol AD, Johanson AJ, Blizzard RM. Short stature associated with normal growth hormone and decreased somatomedin-C concentrations: Response to exogenous growth hormone. Pediatrics 71: 576–580, 1983.

19. Gertner JM, Genel M, Gianfredi SP, Hintz RL, Rosenfeld RG, Tamborlane WV, Wilson DM. Prospective clinical trial of human growth hormone in short children without growth hormone deficiency. J. Pediatr. 104:172–176, 1984.

Questions

1. Are there psychological hazards to the manipulations involved in treating a patient like this with injections of GH?
2. What psychological benefits might accrue if this patient had a significant improvement in growth rate while being treated with GH?
3. What risks to psychological well-being might occur if his growth response does not improve with treatment?

Comments: Brian Stabler*

Potential Psychological Risks in Growth Hormone
Therapy

Whatever else parents may wish for their child, they have the common expectation that the child will grow in stature. Therefore, when a child is brought for assessment of suspected growth failure, it is important to assess not only the presenting problem, but also the reasons why the assessment is being sought. For example, delay in growth may be seen by some families as reflecting a serious, possibly life-threatening problem, whereas others may view it as a social embarrassment, perhaps representing inadequate parental care. Perceptions of what might be the cause of growth failure, as well as what its effects are on life experiences, contribute to the potential psychological risks of treating with GH.

Three issues often arise as psychological factors in considering patients for GH therapy. First, is the consideration of therapy based solely on concern about growth, or is it possible that the patient is being subtly rejected as unacceptable by the parents? If stature is deemed unacceptable, it may follow that other personal qualities such as temperament, intelligence, or athletic ability are also included. Children with chronic medical conditions may be viewed by their parents as unsatisfactory for a variety of reasons, many of which may be entirely unconscious (1). Second, expectations of treatment outcome are subject

*University of North Carolina School of Medicine, Chapel Hill, North Carolina.

to distortion, misinterpretation, or misunderstanding. We did a recent study that showed that parents of growth-delayed children overestimated significantly the effects expected of GH therapy (2). As a result parents may respond negatively when such unrealistic expectations are not fulfilled. Third, for many short children the prospect of undergoing GH injections may not be perceived in as positive a fashion as their parents perceive it. Studies have shown that many short children undergo psychologically painful readjustment to increases in height, particularly if the change is only from the 3rd to the 10th or 15th percentile on growth charts (3). In addition, it is known that children understand the nature and meaning of illness and medical therapy in different ways, depending on their developmental stage (4). Thus it is possible that children may be unwilling or uninformed participants in a treatment that holds long-term psychological implications.

Potential Psychological Benefits of Growth Hormone Therapy

Although retrospective surveys have reported a general level of patient satisfaction with GH treatment, there is as yet little empirical evidence that specific psychological benefits are associated with increased growth velocity. Possible benefits to undertaking GH therapy include three elements: reducing patient and family frustration, parent and patient education, and possible enhancement of patient self-esteem.

In most cases children are referred for evaluation of their GH problem only after an extended period of observation by a pediatrician or general practitioner (5). The ensuing observation period necessary to establish growth velocity may delay diagnosis. Treatment of growth problems is necessarily a time-consuming process. One of the benefits of beginning assessment or treatment is the reduction of tension, frustration, and confusion in the family and the child. Uncertainty about the diagnosis, anxiety over the possible financial implications of undertaking long-term therapy, and the sense of helplessness and frustration brought by protracted inactivity can all be reduced as intervention, albeit only initial assessment, gets under way.

Another, often unrecognized, benefit of beginning the assessment of a growth problem is its contribution to the family and patient understanding of what the growth delay means and what may be expected in the future. Many families fail to recognize their child's slow rate of growth for a considerable time. When the problem is first recognized, the possible causes and the treatment options are not clear. Many parents become confused, particularly if they hear conflicting opinions from different sources. Such confusion can aid unhealthy denial that a problem exists. The evaluation process will usually uncover these ambiguities, anxieties, and uncertainties, and in so doing clarify and redirect family and patient understanding of what is happening.

The psychological effect of being smaller than agemates leads to social isolation, emotional immaturity, poor body image, and lowered self-esteem (6,7). Although few studies have examined the psychological effect of GH therapy, several retrospective patient surveys have been published recently. Mitchell et al. followed 58 patients treated over a 25-year period. Of these, 64% were satisfied with the outcome of treatment, although measures of self-concept showed significantly lower ratings than normal (8). Holmes, Karlsson, and Thompson studied a group of 47 short children of various diagnoses and found that psychological adjustment declined in early adolescence and as many as 25% of the group repeated a grade in school (9). Dean et al. reviewed the adjustment of 116 patients after GH treatment and found that 85% reported that lack of stature was not a social or psychological problem. However, 73% still lived with parents at a mean age of 25 years (10). Clopper's group similarly found that 33% of their patients were living independent of their parents in young adulthood (11). Rosenfeld et al. demonstrated positive social effects in adolescent boys treated with low doses of testosterone (12). Descriptive studies suggest that the short-term effect of increased growth velocity may be enhanced self-image, improved self-esteem and confidence, and an increase in interpersonal peer contacts.

Psychological Aspects of Perceived Treatment "Failure"

Relative treatment "failure" may occur when the expected outcome of treatment does not emerge (13). "Failure" is defined by what the patient or family hopes for or expects from therapy, not necessarily by medical realities. Growth delay is not readily characterized as a chronic disease, such as epilepsy or asthma, and thus is not susceptible to the patient's perception of being "cured." Depending upon the degree of reality the patient's and family's expectations contain, in order of severity the psychological risks may entail the following consequences:

1. At the very least both patient and family may express disappointment at the effects of treatment. This may occur early in treatment and reflect a need to clarify treatment goals for patient and family. Usually such reactions are responsive to physician reassurance.

2. Continued overconcern on the part of a parent during treatment may signal that issues of responsibility for the cause of the problem are still unanswered. Self-blame or guilt may also occur when few signs of increase in growth velocity are evident or when the child responds negatively to the repeated injections. Sometimes such problems are brought about by previously undetected family stresses such as marital discord (1). Disagreements over the continuation of treatment or over who should administer injections may be evident.

3. On occasion a child may feel responsible for "failing" to meet parental expectations for growth, attributing blame to himself, leading to parent–child alienation (14). Children with chronic medical conditions frequently see themselves as being to blame for their condition (15). When such a condition cannot be eliminated, as in the case of diabetes or epilepsy, the patient develops a sense of personal failure. Most common is a feeling of having disappointed significant adults who, in the child's perception, expect him to become well again. If this feeling continues unabated, it can have significant consequences for psychological health.

4. One such consequence commonly associated with problems of body image is diminished self-esteem. Failure to be satisfied with one's physical appearance is a significant factor in shaping a negative self-image (16). Unhappiness with body image leads to anxiety or sadness, particularly if the child

feels rejected or inferior because of his failure to grow. If growth rate does not improve in response to treatment, disappointment may become a more serious and pervasive concern with self-image, feelings of hopelessness may appear, and attempts to compensate for such feelings can include academic failure, acting out through anger or bravado, or withdrawal into passivity or regression (14). Clearly, these are more serious threats to psychological adjustment and should be considered a signal for intervention.

5. Finally, the most serious risk in relation to treatment failure is that the patient will become depressed clinically. Rotnem and colleagues found that a high percentage of their patients showed clinical signs of depression within one year of starting GH treatment (13). Drotar's group reported that the most prominent psychological weakness evident in growth-delayed children was a low tolerance for frustration, a problem also frequently seen in depressed children (17).

The growth-delayed child should be viewed as psychologically vulnerable and be observed closely while in treatment (18). If significant psychological stress is noted, regardless of the "success" or "failure" of medical treatment, appropriate psychotherapy should be instituted.

References

1. Burton L. The Family Life of Sick Children. Routledge & Kegan Paul, Boston, 1974.

2. Grew RS, Stabler B, Williams RW, Underwood LE. Facilitating patient understanding in the treatment of growth delay. Clin. Pediatr. 22:685, 193.

3. Money J. Counseling: Syndromes of statural hypoplasia and hyperplasia, precocity and delay. In Endocrine and Genetic Diseases of Childhood and Adolescence, 2nd ed., Gardner LI, ed., Saunders, Philadelphia, 1975.

4. Piaget J. The Child's Conception of the World. Littlefield, Adams & Co., Totowa, NJ, 1976.

5. Underwood LE. Growth hormone treatment for short children. J. Pediatr. 104:237, 1984.

6. Steinhausen HC, Stahnke N. Negative impact of growth hormone deficiency on psychological functioning in dwarfed children and adolescents. Eur. J. Pediatr. 126:263, 1977.

7. Spencer RF, Raft DD. Adaptation and defenses in hypopituitary dwarfs. Psychosomatics 15:35, 1974.

8. Mitchell CM, Johanson AJ, Joyce S, Libber S, Plotnick L, Migeon CJ, Blizzard RM. Psychosocial impact of long-term growth hormone therapy. In Slow Grows the Child, Stabler B, Underwood LE, eds., Erlbaum, Hillsdale, NJ, 1986.

9. Holmes CS, Karlsson JA, Thompson RG. Longitudinal evaluation of behavior patterns in children with short stature. In Slow Grows the Child, Stabler B, Underwood LE, eds., Erlbaum, Hillsdale, NJ, 1986.

10. Dean HJ, McTaggart TL, Fish DG, Friesen HG. Long-term social follow-up of growth hormone deficient adults treated with growth hormone during childhood. In Slow Grows the Child, Stabler B, Underwood LE, eds., Erlbaum, Hillsdale, NJ, 1986.

11. Clopper RR, MacGillivray MH, Mazur T, Voorhess ML, Mills BJ. Post-treatment follow-up of growth hormone deficient patients: Psychosocial status. In Slow Grows the Child, Stabler B, Underwood LE, eds., Erlbaum, Hillsdale, NJ, 1986.

12. Rosenfeld RG, Northcraft GB, Hintz RL. A prospective, randomized study of testosterone treatment of constitutional delay of growth and development in male adolescents. Pediatrics 69:681–687, 1982.

13. Rotnem D, Cohen DJ, Hintz RL, Genel M. Psychological sequelae of relative "treatment failure" for children receiving human growth hormone replacement. J. Am. Acad. Child Psychiat. 18:505, 1979.

14. Rotnem D. Size versus age: Ambiguities in parenting short statured children. In Slow Grows the Child, Stabler B, Underwood LE, eds., Erlbaum, Hillsdale, NJ. 1986.

15.. Mattsson A. Long-term physical illness in childhood: A challenge to psychosocial adaptation. Pediatrics 50:801, 1972.

16. Alport GW. Pattern and Growth in Personality. Holt, Rinehart & Winston, New York, 1961.

17. Drotar D, Owens R, Gothold J. Personality adjustment of children and
     adolescents with hypopituitarism. Child Psychiat. Hum. Dev. 11:59,
     1980.
18. Ad Hoc Committee on Growth Hormone Usage. Growth hormone treat-
     ment of children with short stature. Pediatrics 72, 6:891, 1983.

Editors' Note

This patient was treated in an experimental protocol with National
Hormone and Pituitary Program growth hormone (0.1 mg/kg three
times weekly) for 6 months. His growth rate during this period was 8.7
cm/year.

CASE 3

The patient, a white boy, was referred at 8.7 years for evaluation of
extreme short stature. He was the 3068-g product of a normal 40-week
pregnancy and a normal delivery. He had a normal infancy and was
believed to be growing well until 12–18 months of age. After this, his
growth slowed and by 3 years of age his height was well below the 3rd
percentile. His general health has been excellent and his psychological
adjustment is said to be good.

His mother is 144.5 cm (57 inches) tall and his father is 157 cm
(62 inches). Both are normally proportioned and have no history of
chronic illnesses. The paternal grandmother and grandfather are 163
and 165 cm, respectively; the maternal grandmother and grandfather
are 150 and 157 cm, respectively. a 4½-year-old sister is said to be at
the 50th percentile for height.

On physical examination this boy was small but normally proportioned. His height was 103.2 cm (height age, 4.3 years; Figure 7) and
weight was 17.7 kg (weight age, 4.7 years). Arm span was 101.5 cm.
There were no abnormal physical findings.

Determinations of serum electrolytes, enzymes, and renal function tests revealed no abnormality. Urinalysis was normal. Total serum
thyroxine was 9.7 μg/dl, and plasma Sm-C/IGF-I was 1.6 U/ml.
Bone age x-rays of the hand and wrist were read as 6.5 years.

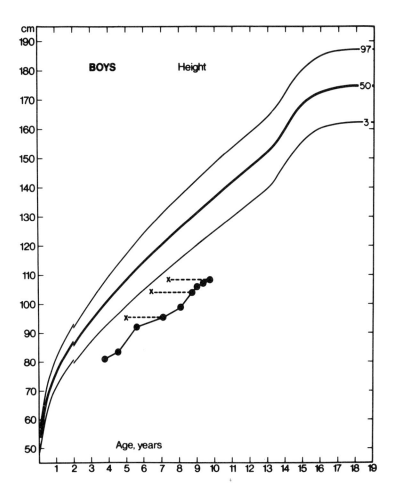

Figure 7. Growth chart for the boy discussed in case 3.

At 9.0 years his serum growth hormone rose to 30 ng/ml 75 minutes after taking 0.1 mg clonidine orally, and to 25 ng/ml following L-dopa. Skull x-rays revealed a normal sella turcica. Height was 105.3 cm (interval growth rate, 6.1 cm/yr) and weight was 18.5 kg.

At 9.3 his height was 106.8 cm (growth rate, 5.3 cm/year) and weight was 19.3 kg. At 9.7 years his height was 108.7 cm (interval growth rate, 4.9 cm/year) and weight was 21.0 kg. Bone age was 7.5 years.

Questions

1. The patient's height is well below the 3rd percentile. Should he be treated with GH?
2. If he were experiencing psychological problems, would you be more inclined to treat with GH?
3. If this patient's parents were of average size and he had been small for gestational size, would he be a candidate for GH therapy?
4. Is there any way to foretell a response to GH therapy?

Comments: Selna L. Kaplan*

Since 7 years of age, and during the past year, this boy has grown at a rate of 5.5 cm/year. The slight variations in growth rate observed during the 3–4 month intervals are not significantly different when compared to his overall yearly rate. His predicted height of 148–150 cm is appropriate for his family, in which there is genetic short stature.

Based on our data, 70% of children who have a subnormal growth rate (less than 5 cm/year) and a 2-year or more retardation in bone age would have an acceleration in growth rate when treated with hGH. In those with a "normal" growth rate (5 cm or more per year) and a retarded bone age, only 5–10% show a beneficial effect of hGH treatment (Table 2).

I would not treat this child with GH and I would not be influenced

---

*University of California at San Francisco School of Medicine, San Francisco, California.

Table 2. Comparison of Responders and Nonresponders to
Growth Hormone in Short Normal Children

Subgroup	CA (years)	BA (years)	HV less than 3rd percentile for BA
Responders	7.1 ± 1.2	−3.7 ± 0.6	5/6
Nonresponders	11.9 ± 0.9	−2.0 ± 0.3	1/8
p	0.01	0.02	0.02

Source: Ref. 9.

by psychological problems. We do not resolve the psychological problems if we recommend GH therapy and no benefit is derived. We need
to emphasize that the short stature will not be resolved for many years,
even if he did have an acceleration in growth rate. Further, the beneficial effect of GH therapy on final height may result in only 1–2 inches
of added height. Further studies are needed in children with genetic
short stature.

GH therapy in small-for-dates children has not been shown to
improve final height. Further studies are needed on such patients.

Although I know of no laboratory test that will foretell the response to GH therapy, I believe that a subnormal growth rate and
delayed bone age may be predictive of a response to GH therapy in
some instances.

Comments: Barbara M. Lippe*

The patient has a family history, medical history, physical examination, laboratory studies, and growth pattern consistent with a combination of constitutional growth delay and genetic short stature. Length of
gestation was normal and there was no evidence of a significant intra-

---

*University of California at Los Angeles School of Medicine, Los Angeles, Califor-
nia.

uterine problem. His abnormal growth deceleration was said to have occurred after 12–18 months of age and the accompanying growth chart indicates that his growth after age 3½ years shows no further significant deceleration. Parenthetically, I suspect that his growth was either at a very low percentile for the first year or that abnormal or excessive deceleration occurred at or before 12 months, to account for his stature at 3½ years. If the latter is the case, his growth pattern would be consistent with the data of Smith and co-workers who suggest that "lagging-down" or downchanneling to one's targeted midparental height channel occurs in midinfancy (mean age to reach new channel is 13 months) and is complete by 2 years (1).

The data of Horner and co-workers indicate that the pattern of growth most frequently associated with constitutional delay is that of an abnormally rapid deceleration until age 3 years, followed by a normal growth velocity thereafter (2). Thus this patient's loss in height between ages 2 and 3 is consistent with this diagnosis and is supported later by his delay in bone age. Correcting his height for the 2-year delays in bone age places him into a channel consistent with that of his targeted midparental height of 157 cm. This delay in growth is likely to translate into pubertal delay and might present another question of management independent of stature.

The GH responses to provocative stimuli are normal and preclude classical GH deficiency. While neither the plasma Sm-C/IGF-I assay method nor the age-adjusted normal range is given, the value is consistent with normal GH secretion.

Thus, three key questions are posed: 1.) Should a child like this be treated with GH? 2.) Should any child with genetic short stature be treated with GH? 3.) Is there any way to foretell a response to GH treatment?

In response to the first two questions I would ask the following: 1.) Do we believe that GH administered as a pharmacological agent can increase safely the height of genetically short children: 2.) Are we willing to support a clinical study to answer this question? 3.) Are we willing to accept the medical, social, financial, and psychological risks that we may encounter in the effort to answer these questions?

The data available currently are insufficient to answer the first question. That is, only a limited number of reports address the question of whether treatment with GH in the doses available previously will increase adult stature, and these are limited to patients with GH deficiency. The results of these studies suggest that fewer than half of the patients reach their targeted midparental adult stature (3,4). Recognizing the limitations of these studies, the data on the heights of pituitary-dependent acromegalic giants are often used to support the contention that GH can increase genetic height potential. The use of these patients as models may be flawed, because most of the pituitary giants who have had complete endocrine evaluations have gonadotropin deficiency as a consequence of their pituitary tumor. It is possible, therefore, that their increased period of growth was related partly to the lack of pubertal gonadal hormones promoting epiphysial fusion.

The second question addresses the commitment of the medical community and of society to support the studies necessary to determine the long-term effects of GH. It is easy to imagine that a physician might be willing to ask a child and family to commit to a limited course of high-dose GH treatment. The results of this experiment might not translate to later growth, and one can foresee that the effects of immediate gratification could prevail and follow-up studies might not be done. It is harder to assess the willingness of the physician to support the participation of a patient in a long-term (3–5 year) trial that determines whether ultimate height is greater. I believe that such studies are needed and will require patient and physician education before they can be done.

The third original question was whether there was a way to foretell a response to GH treatment. The answer to this is probably not. That does not mean that we should settle for this. The biochemical, physiological, and clinical criteria we hoped would provide answers (i.e., Sm-C/IGF-I response to short-term treatment, GH response to stimuli, or growth rate and bone age delay) are not sufficiently sensitive. We could argue that only a clinical trial is a predictor of response. However, this argument is limited to the time of the trial and does not necessarily predict long-term efficacy. Therefore, the short-term clinical trial may be our only method to assess the nonresponder, but long-term trials coupled with laboratory methods that are not yet developed will be necessary to determine who will benefit ultimately.

Finally, there are several psychological and philosophical issues raised by this case. We need to ask when (and how) the psychological stress experienced by a child should become a part of the process of choosing a specific therapy. If short stature creates psychological stress, should the treatment focus on accelerating growth or should it be directed at help in dealing with self-esteem? If a trial of GH is unsuccessful, the child may perceive that the physician believed that his short stature was a condition worthy of treatment, but that he failed because the treatment failed. In addition, in a child as short as the one described, short-term growth acceleration is unlikely to result in growth sufficient to produce an effect that the child's peers will notice. Therefore, one would be using an experimental treatment for what is primarily a placebo effect (showing the child that someone is trying to help him or her). Again, this transmits the message that short stature needs to be helped. Finally, if short-term growth acceleration is the objective, the patient described would likely experience equally good acceleration with low-dose androgen. I believe that while GH is in the experimental stages, it should be used in children who are psychologically stable and capable of accepting a program designed to answer the question of growth hormone's ultimate efficacy. Anabolic steroids might be better if only short-term treatment is planned.

We should also ask which kind of short stature we should attempt to treat. Is genetic short stature a more or less compelling condition than uncomplicated intrauterine growth retardation? In terms of population genetics, genetic short stature will not be altered by therapy, in that the offspring of the treated individual will have the same "short" genes (the creation of a somewhat taller parent might influence the choice of mate, but the mate may have been "treated" also). Therefore, we could be putting offspring in an even more difficult position than their parents perceived they were in; that is, being short but having tall parents. These children would then also be candidates for treatment. This would suggest that the patient with intrauterine growth retardation is a more logical candidate. If he or she has normal genetic potential, successful treatment would facilitate choice of mate of similar height resulting in offspring who would not need treatment. I believe that patients of this type should be studied and treated. One problem with treating such patients is that intrauterine growth retardation has many causes; therefore, an extensive commitment of resources would be needed to obtain interpretable data on long-term efficacy.

References

1. Smith DW, Troug W, Rogers JE, et al. Shifting linear growth during infancy: Illustration of genetic factors in growth from fetal life through infancy. J. Pediatr. 89:225, 1986.

2. Horner JM, Thorsson AV, Hintz RL. Growth deceleration patterns in children with constitutional short stature: An aid to diagnosis. Pediatrics 62:529, 1978.

3. Burns EC, Tanner JM, Preece MA, Cameron N. Final height and pubertal development in 55 children with idiopathic growth hormone deficiency, treated for between 2 and 15 years with human growth hormone. Eur. J. Pediatr. 137:155, 1981.

4. Joss E, Zuppinger, K, Schwarz HP, Roten H. Final height of patients with pituitary growth failure and changes in growth variables after long term hormonal therapy. Pediatr. Res. 17:676, 1983.

Comments: Robert M. Blizzard*

The boy's diagnosis may be genetic short stature. Some element of constitutional delay is present since the bone age is 7.5 years at a chronological age of 9.7 years. Using Tanner's graphs that take into account midparental heights, this boy falls more than 3 SD below the 50th percentile. His predicted height using the Bayley-Pinneau prediction table is 154 cm. Assuming that his bone age would be read similarly by the TW2 method, his predicted adult height is 148 cm. Therefore, there may be factors contributing to his short stature other than genetic short stature and constitutional delay. The cause of these, if present, is not apparent.

This is the type of patient who should be admitted into a protocol to test his growth response to GH injections. The GH in his serum following stimulation by clonidine should be determined by the usual radioimmunoassay for GH, by the radioreceptor assay for GH utilizing IM-9 cells, and by the radioimmunometric assay. Ratios of these should be determined and compared subsequently with the ratios of other patients who will be entered into the same protocol. With such data we

*University of Virginia School of Medicine, Charlottesville, Virginia.

could come up eventually with a way to predict patients who might respond to GH therapy.

The dosage of GH that I would recommend is 5.7 mg or 11.4 U/week. This calculation is derived using his body weight of approximately 19 kg and a dose of 0.1 mg/kg three times a week. I would prefer to treat him daily because it is logical that daily injections might increase growth rate more than when GH is given three times weekly. This schedule would better simulate the normal pulsatility pattern of GH secretion. Unpublished data from our laboratory indicates that GH disappears from blood within 12–16 hours after intramuscular injection. Therefore, with an injection only three times a week there are many hours during the week when serum GH cannot be measured.

Even in the absence of psychological problems of significant degree, I believe this boy should be placed on treatment in a protocol unless he resists adamantly. I cannot predict whether his growth rate will increase or whether he will have increased adult height. On the basis of the Sm-C/IGF-I determination, which is in the upper range of normal, I would be less inclined to think that this boy would benefit than if his Sm-C/IGF-I was in the lower range of normal or was low. This statement is made on the basis of such reports as that of Rudman et al. (1), although I am aware that Van Vliet et al. (2) have reported that Sm-C/IGF-I determinations are not good predictors for growth when GH is given to non-GH short children.

If this boy's parents were of average size and he had been small for gestational age, I would be inclined to enter him into a protocol for GH therapy. This decision is made on the basis of data of Foley et al. Twelve patients with low birth weights and birth lengths for gestational age were treated with GH for 5–18 months. Significant delay in skeletal maturation was present in all but one patient. Eight patients who were 7 years of age or younger at the time of treatment and who had pretreatment growth rates of approximately 5 cm/year increased their growth rate to at least twice the pretreatment growth rate. In six of the eight (75%) the growth rates on treatment were improved by 3.5 cm or more per year. Among those patients who received their initial course of growth hormone therapy in a dose of 2 IU or more/m^2/day, five of eight (62.5%) more than doubled their pretreatment growth rates. Seven of the eight (88%) increased their pretreatment growth rates by more than

3.5 cm/year during therapy. Unfortunately, no predictors of response were found, including nitrogen balance. Sm-C/IGF-I determinations were not done, and radioreceptor and radioimmunometric assays were not available.

The cost of treatment in such a patient is of importance. In the article by Foley et al. (3) the dosage used was approximately 14 U/m² or 14 U/28 kg week. At $20/unit, this could cost $14,560/year for a 28-kg patient. This is comparable to the cost paid by many parents to treat their GH-deficient children. In my opinion, studies of patients such as the one described in this case history certainly should be done to evaluate whether GH can increase growth rate and to determine whether it will increase ultimate height.

References

1. Rudman D, Kuetner MH, Blackston RD, Cushman RA, Bain RP, Patterson JH. Children with normal-variant short stature: Treatment with human growth hormone for six months. N. Engl. J. Med. 305:23, 1981.

2. Van Vliet G, Styne DM, Kaplan SL, Grumbach MM. Growth hormone treatment for short stature. N. Engl. J. Med. 309:1016–1022, 1983.

3. Foley TP Jr, Thompson RG, Shaw M, Baghdassarian A, Nissley SP, Blizzard RM. Growth responses to human growth hormone in patients with intrauterine growth retardation. J. Pediatr. 84:635, 1974.

Questions

1. What ethical issues should be considered in treating a patient such as the one described?

2. Is it ethical to treat short children if parents demand GH therapy for their short child but the physician is uncertain whether it will stimulate short-term or long-term growth rate, have any beneficial effect on adult height, or not have adverse side effects?

Comments: Eric T. Juengst*

Until now, the pressing ethical issue in GH therapy has been the problem of distributing the limited supplies of pituitary GH among those who needed it. With the development and approval of biosynthetic GH, however, that problem has moved a long way toward being solved. The scientists and clinicians involved in resolving this problem can be proud of their accomplishment. On the other hand, solving ethical problems rarely decreases the overall number of problems to be solved. My purpose here is to review some of the questions the biosynthetic solution to the GH rationing problem can raise for clinicians faced with cases like Case 3. Four sets of considerations seem especially relevant to this case.

Benefiting the Patient

One of the oldest moral themes in medicine concerns the duty of physicians to benefit their patients (1). The first set of ethical questions one might consider with Case 3 reflects that tradition. The benefit that physicians usually try to provide cluster around the cure of disease, the restoration of compromised function, and the relief of suffering. Will GH therapy allow us to provide any of these benefits to the patient in Case 3? In what sense is this patient diseased, disabled, or suffering to begin with?

The answer to the question brings up an important point about medicine: what we count as a medical problem is often influenced by what we value as a society (2). However, that influence can work in different ways, with different implications for ethical treatment. For example, the patient's stature might be counted as a handicap simply out of a cultural prejudice against short people. In that case, combating the prejudice seems a more appropriate response than treating the child. Alternatively, the child may face some real disabilities, but only within the context of the environment our biased society has built around him. Here, the justification for treatment will increase pri-

---

*University of California at San Francisco School of Medicine, San Francisco, California.

marily with the difficulty of adapting the patient's environment to his needs. Finally, society's attitudes toward stature may cause the patient real psychological suffering. If GH treatment could alleviate or prevent that suffering, its benefits would be clearer still.

The *ethical* challenge in deciding whether treatment is indicated in this case, in sum, is to determine whether the patient could benefit more from changes we can reasonably expect to make in his stature or from changes we can reasonably expect to make in the environment that makes his stature a problem. This challenge makes our questions about the efficacy of GH treatment particularly ethically important (3). As confidence in the power of the therapy to prevent psychological suffering and restore normal development weakens, the obligation to benefit the patient through other means grows stronger.

Respecting Patients' Preferences

Uncertainty over the efficacy of GH therapy raises other ethical considerations in treating Case 3. An axiom of modern clinical ethics is that as medical uncertainty increases, it becomes correspondingly more important to share treatment decisions with the affected patient (4). In effect, clinical judgments like a decision to use GH in Case 3 are "quality of life" judgments made on the patient's behalf. They imply an evaluation of the patient's life-experience and the risks that are worth taking to improve it. Whenever possible, our respect for patients' stakes in these judgments demands that they be able to contribute to them.

With Case 3, the clinician's duty to involve the patient in treatment decisions raises two questions, both concerned with the fact that the patient is a child. First, is the patient mature enough to participate helpfully in a decision regarding GH therapy? His ability to appreciate the choices before him, rather than his age alone, should be decisive in determining how to weigh his views. In any case, it may be useful to explore the nature of his current successful adjustment to his stature to see what it implies about the relative worth of treatment to him.

Second, what about the parents' preferences? If the parents demand GH therapy, is the clinician obligated to provide it? Interestingly, despite individuals' moral power to *refuse* medically indicated treatment, patients have little authority to demand treatment against a physician's better judgment, and patients' parents even less. Where there is no relative benefit to treatment, the basic medical ethical principle of beneficence provides an outer limit to the physician's duty to respect patient's preferences for care. Given the uncertainties in cases like Case 3, more indications for treatment than simply a parental request seem required before it would be ethical to proceed.

Weighing Benefits and Burdens

Uncertainty about the effects of GH therapy raises a third set of moral considerations relevant to Case 3: questions about the possible harms this treatment might inflict. First, there are questions about the possible side effects of treating short-normal children with GH (5). But perhaps less obvious, the psychological burden of the treatment itself should also be considered. If the benefits of GH therapy are unclear, the psychological costs of associating the patient's short stature with a series of intramuscular injectons and hospital visits seems all too clear: he will definitely know that someone thinks he has a medical problem (6). As a reflection of the reverse of the duty to benefit—the duty to "do no harm"—these potential harms also have to be factored into the decisions. In Case 3, one would want particularly to weigh the costs of treatment to the patient's current psychological health against the psychological problems we might reasonably expect the treatment to prevent in the future.

Burdens to Others

A final set of considerations involves the burdens that treating this patient will place on others. Here the focus shifts from Case 3 to the future cases for which Case 3 helps set the "standard of care." One concern here is to set a clinical precedent that will discourage the *abuse* of the hormone, without the necessity of regulating GH as a "controlled substance" (7). More generally, the point here is to try to curb treatment practices that merely reinforce the sociocultural roots of the problem they are designed to address. Might the casual "medical" use of GH by those who can afford the treatment, by linking height even more closely to other socially valuable traits like wealth and health, merely lead to the exacerbation of the general bias against short stature (8)? These considerations, though less weighty than those focused on the patient at hand, may be decisive in some borderline cases.

This outline only hints at the complexity of the ethical considerations that will arise in deciding to treat patients like Case 3. It does, however, provide a scheme for thinking through the issues. In short, one works through such decisions by considering what will benefit the patient within the constraints of the patient's wishes and to the extent that foreseeable harm to the patient and others is minimized.

References

1. Nelson LJ. Primum utilis esse: The primacy of usefulness in medicine. Yale J. Biol. Med. 51:655–667, 1978.

2. Engelhardt HT. Ideology and etiology, J. Med. Philos. 1:256–267, 1976.

3. Ad Hoc Committee on Growth Hormone Usage. Growth hormone in the treatment of children with short stature. Pediatrics 72:891–894, 1984.

4. The President's Commission for the Study of Ethical Problems in Medicine and Biomedical and Behavioral Research. Making Health Care Decisions: The Ethical and Legal Implications of Informed Consent in the Patient-Practitioner Relationship. U.S. Government Printing Office, Washington, 1982.

5. Underwood LE. Growth hormone treatment for short children. Pediatrics 104:237–238, 1984.

6. Benjamin M, Muyskens J, Saenger P. Short children, anxious parents: Is growth hormone the answer? The Hastings Center Report 14:5–9, 1984.

7. Taylor W. Synthetic hGH should be classified as a controlled substance to prevent abuse. Gen. Eng. News 6:4,37, March 1986.

8. Murray T. Human growth hormone and abuse potential, Gen. Eng. News 4:6,27, May/June 1984.

9. Van Vliet G, Styne DM, Kaplan SL, Grumbach MM. Growth hormone treatment of short stature. N. Engl. J. Med. 309:1016–1022, 1983.

8

Growth Hormone Therapy in Turner Syndrome

RON G. ROSENFELD
and RAYMOND L. HINTZ
Stanford University School of Medicine
Stanford, California

I. GROWTH IN TURNER SYNDROME

In his original description of the syndrome that now bears his name, Henry Turner characterized the requisite clinical features as sexual infantilism, webbing of the neck, and cubitus valgus (1). Although short stature was described in several of his seven patients, Turner did not consider it a prerequisite for the diagnosis of Turner syndrome. In this regard, it is of historical interest to note that Turner actually treated some of his original patients with anterior pituitary growth hormone (presumably a crude bovine preparation) and reported the results to be unsatisfactory.

Table 1.   Final Adult Height in Turner Syndrome

Study	Mean adult height (cm)	Range (cm)
Park et al. (3)	142.0	131.2–167.0
Brook et al. (4)	142.5	131.5–150.5
Lev-Ran (5)	143.2	134.0–153.0
Sybert (6)	146.3	136.0–156.0
Ranke et al. (7)	146.8	

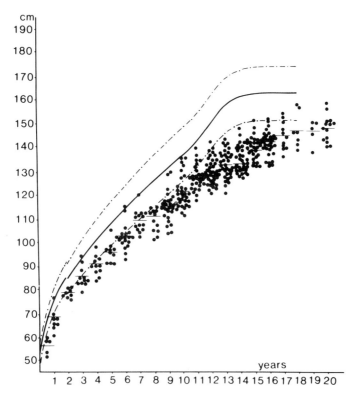

Figure 1A.   Height in patients with Turner syndrome compared to the normal range. (From Ref. 7.)

Subsequent large reviews of the clinical phenotype of Turner syndrome found short stature to be an almost universal feature. Palmer and Reichmann reported that all of 110 patients had short stature, regardless of karyotype (2). Similarly, Park and co-workers found short stature in 100% of 45,X patients and 95% of non-45,X individuals (3). Studies of Turner syndrome patients from around the world have reported mean final adult height to range from 142.0 to 146.8 cm (3–7) (Table 1).

Figure 1 presents the results of 384 single measurements of height in 150 German children with Turner syndrome and compares these

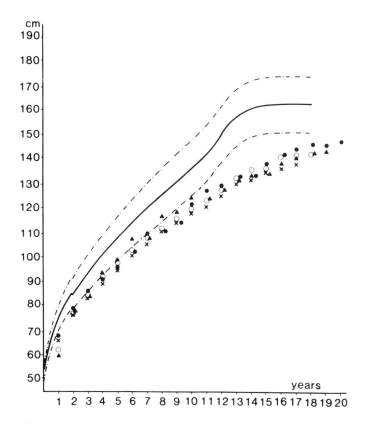

Figure 1B. Mean height in patients with Turner syndrome observed by different investigators. *Key*: ○ Brook et al.; × Lenko et al.; ▲ Pelz et al.; ● Ranke et al. (From Ref. 7.)

results to data from other European studies (7). As can be seen, considerable variability in final adult height exists. In general, children progressively deviate from the normal height percentiles until approximately 14 years of age, followed by a gradual approach toward the normal percentiles because of delayed epiphyseal maturation. Final adult heights frequently are not reached until 19 years of age, and some individuals continue growing into their twenties. It is also important to note that the younger the patient, the greater the possibility that her

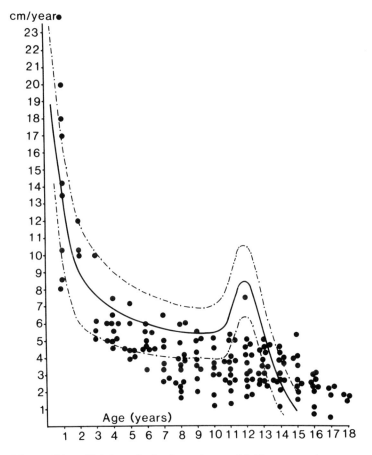

Figure 2A. Height velocity in patients with Turner syndrome compared to the normal range. (From Ref. 7.)

height may actually fall within the normal height percentiles for age. As a result, girls without many classic Turner stigmata may not present with short stature until late childhood or adolescence, when growth failure often is observed in combination with delayed puberty.

Height velocity data from this same cohort of German and European subjects are shown in Figure 2 (7). On the basis of these observations, Ranke and co-workers identified several distinct growth phases

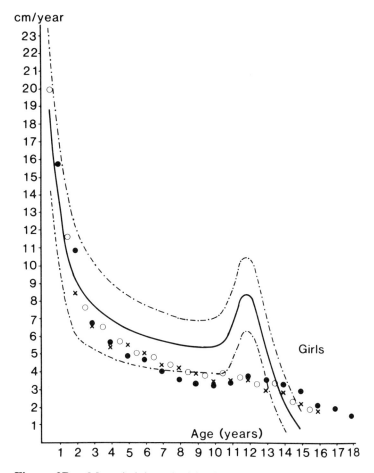

Figure 2B. Mean height velocities in patients with Turner syndrome observed by different investigators. See Figure 1B for key.

in children with Turner syndrome: 1.) a tendency toward mild intra-uterine growth failure, with mean birth weights and lengths of 2828 g and 48.3 cm, respectively; 2.) normal mean height gain from birth until approximately 3 years of age; 3.) progressive declines in height velocity and deviation from normal height percentiles until approximately 14 years of age; and 4.) a prolonged adolescent growth phase, characterized by partial return toward normal height (7).

The etiology of growth failure in Turner syndrome remains unclear. Although several cases of simultaneous GH deficiency and Turner syndrome have been reported (8–10), the overwhelming majority of children with Turner syndrome respond to provocative testing with serum GH levels exceeding 7 ng/ml. Nevertheless, the possibility of a partial defect in GH secretion has been supported by the observation of Laczi et al. (11) that peak GH levels following insulin-induced hypoglycemia averaged only 14.9 ng/ml in patients with Turner syndrome, compared to 54.3 ng/ml in age-matched controls (11). Ross et al. reported that older girls (9–20 years) with Turner syndrome had significantly reduced mean 24-hour GH levels, peak amplitudes, and peak frequencies (12). These findings cannot, however, explain the presence of growth failure in many younger girls with Turner syndrome. Finally, this same report documented significantly reduced plasma somatomedin C (Sm-C) levels in Turner patients between the ages of 6 and 12 years, and Cuttler et al. reported significantly reduced Sm-C levels in patients between 11 and 16 years of age (13). In our experience in the Genentech Collaborative Study, 37% of subjects had baseline Sm-C levels below the 95% confidence limit of age-matched controls (14). In the older age groups, decreased plasma Sm-C levels were especially common, perhaps reflecting the lack of spontaneous puberty. Studies performed on fibroblasts derived from subjects with Turner syndrome have demonstrated normal Sm-C binding and responsiveness, making the possibility of end-organ resistance to somatomedin unlikely (15).

Because of the high incidence of skeletal abnormalities in Turner syndrome, it has been suggested that the etiology of short stature in this condition is not hormonal but rather the inevitable result of an inborn skeletal dysplasia. Common bony abnormalities include disproportion of the axial segments with abnormal upper-to-lower segment ratios, hypoplasia of the cervical vertebrae, abnormalities of the trochlear head, Madelung's deformity, short metacarpals, micrognathia, genu valgum, and scoliosis. Additionally, bones of Turner patients frequently give the radiologic appearance of osteoporosis, which may in fact represent a primary dysplasia rather than demineralization.

II. THERAPY FOR SHORT STATURE IN TURNER SYNDROME: HISTORICAL PERSPECTIVE

Therapy directed primarily at augmentation of growth and final adult height in patients with Turner syndrome has involved three different hormonal approaches: 1.) androgens and anabolic steroids; 2.) estrogens; and 3.) growth hormone. Despite multiple studies of anabolic steroids over the last 20 years, very few controlled, prospective data exist concerning long-term effects of such therapy on final adult height. In general, studies have demonstrated that such agents are successful in stimulating short-term growth, but controversy remains concerning the effect of therapy on eventual adult height. In an uncontrolled, retrospective study, Urban et al. reported that patients treated with oxandrolone, fluoxymesterone, or both were significantly taller as adults than patients treated with estrogen alone (16). Similarly, Lenko et al. treated 25 patients between 9 and 17 years for a minimum of 1 year with fluoxymesterone and reported a general increase in predicted adult height (17). These studies contrast with the report by Sybert that final adult height of Turner patients treated with either oxandrolone or fluoxymesterone did not differ significantly from that of untreated subjects (6).

    In a preliminary study of the effect of various estrogen doses on short-term growth in Turner syndrome, Ross and co-workers studied ulnar growth rates using the Valk device (18). They reported a biphasic effect of estrogen on ulnar growth, with an almost 100% increase in growth observed with an ethinyl estradiol dose of 100 ng/kg/day. Little, if any, growth stimulation was observed at lower or higher estrogen doses. It is important to note that optimal growth was observed at an ethinyl estradiol dosage (100 ng/kg/day) considerably lower than that commonly employed as estrogen replacement for the stimulation of secondary sexual maturation. Nevertheless, the long-term effects of low-dose estrogen on final adult height, as well as its safety in younger girls with Turner syndrome, remain unsettled.

Until recently, limitations in the supply of pituitary-derived hGH have restricted studies on the use of hGH in Turner syndrome, so that most reports have consisted of a small number of patients, typically treated for short periods of time in an uncontrolled manner. While studies by Hutchings et al. (19) and Tzagournis (20) in several girls with Turner syndrome indicated a short-term acceleration of growth velocity, Butenandt (21) reported that doses of hGH up to 36 U/m²/ week did not improve growth rates. Stahnke (22) also reported that hGH was effective in only two of eight girls with Turner syndrome, although the mean chronological age of treated subjects was already 16 years at the initiation of therapy. Rudman et al. studied six patients with Turner syndrome who, over six successive 3-month periods, received no treatment, oxandrolone, hGH, or oxandrolone plus hGH (23). Mean growth rates expressed as centimeters per month were 0.17 for the no-treatment group, 0.27 for oxandrolone, 0.32 for hGH, and 0.63 for combination oxandrolone and hGH.

III. THE GENENTECH COLLABORATIVE STUDY

With the development of recombinant DNA-derived hGH preparations, large-scale studies of the use of hGH in girls with Turner syndrome became feasible. In 1983 a multicenter collaborative study involving 70 patients with Turner syndrome was begun (14). Table 2 lists the participating medical centers and investigators.

Subjects involved in the study ranged in chronological age from 4.7 to 12.4 years, with a mean of 9.3 years. Bone age averaged 8.0 years, with the highest skeletal age being 11.2 years. Of the subjects, 76% had a 45,X karyotype, with the remainder having either mosaicism or a structurally abnormal X chromosome. Patients with any identifiable Y chromosomal material were excluded. All subjects were documented to have a serum GH level of at least 7 ng/ml following

Table 2. Participants in the Genentech
Collaborative Study

Medical center	Investigator(s)
Harbor-UCLA	Jo Anne Brasel
University of Chicago	Stephen Burstein
Cincinnati Children's Hospital	Steven Chernausek
University of Kansas	Wayne Moore
	Teresa Clabots
University of Colorado	Ron Gotlin
UCLA	Barbara Lippe
Mason Clinic	Patrick Mahoney
Cornell	Maria New
	Elizabeth Stoner
Montefiore	Paul Saenger
University of Washington	Virginia Sybert
Stanford	Ron Rosenfeld
	Raymond Hintz
Genentech, Inc.	Ann Johanson
	Joyce Kuntze
	James Frane

provocative testing. Additionally, all subjects were followed for a minimum of 6 months to document pretreatment growth rates. After all eligibility criteria had been met, subjects were assigned to one of four study arms, using a variant of Efron's technique for randomizing and balancing a complex sequential investigation. This was done to assure that all study arms would have similar mean chronological age, bone age, height, weight, growth velocity, and karyotypic patterns.

The four study arms were: 1.) observation; 2.) oxandrolone, 0.125 mg/kg/day orally; 3.) methionyl hGH, 0.125 mg/kg three times a week, administered intramuscularly; and 4.) combination oxandrolone and hGH. Of the 70 randomized subjects, 67 successfully completed the first year of the study.

Prerandomization growth velocity averaged 4.3 ± 1.0 cm/year. In the subsequent year, the observation group grew 3.8 ± 1.0 cm/year. By comparison, the methionyl hGH group grew 6.6 ± 1.2 cm/

year, the oxandrolone group 7.9 ± 1.2 cm/year, and the combination group 9.8 ± 1.4 cm/year. The mean growth rates for each of the various treatment groups were significantly greater than both the control group growth rate and the pretreatment growth rate ($p < .00005$). Additionally, the combination group had a significantly higher growth rate than either oxandrolone or hGH alone ($p < .0005$). These results are summarized in Table 3.

When these data are expressed as standard deviations of growth velocity for girls with Turner syndrome, as published by Ranke, the 1-year growth rates are even more impressive (24) (Table 3). While the observation group had a mean growth velocity of −0.1 SD, the mean growth velocities for the treatment groups were +2.3 (Met-hGH), +3.7 (oxandrolone), and +5.4 (combination).

Plasma Sm-C levels averaged 0.65 ± 0.30 U/ml for the observation group. After 1 year of treatment, plasma Sm-C levels in the hGH group averaged 1.52 ± 0.69 U/ml, while levels in the combination group averaged 1.31 ± 0.59 U/ml. Interestingly, very little rise in Sm-C levels was observed in the oxandrolone group (0.93 ± 0.64 U/ml), despite the fact that children in this group grew at a mean growth rate of 7.9 cm/year.

All treatments resulted in acceleration of skeletal age. Mean 1-year increment in bone age in the observation group was 0.6 year, compared

Table 3. Growth Velocities in Turner Syndrome Subjects

Group	Growth velocity	
	cm/year	Standard deviations[a]
Control	3.8 ± 1.0[b]	−0.1
Met-hGH	6.6 ± 1.2	+2.3
Oxandrolone	7.9 ± 1.0	+3.7
Combination	9.8 ± 1.4	+5.4

[a]Standard deviation of growth velocity for girls with Turner syndrome (24).
[b]Mean ± standard deviation.

to 1.1 years (hGH), 1.3 years (oxandrolone), and 1.6 years (combination). Nevertheless, the increment in height age for the treated patients was so large that the median change in height age-to-bone age ratio ranged from 1.0 to 1.1 for the various treatments, compared to only 0.8 for the observation group. Furthermore, when the Bayley-Pinneau method of height prediction was applied to subjects with a minimum bone age of 6.0 years, all treatment groups showed a significant increase in predicted adult heights: +2.5 cm for hGH or oxandrolone alone, and +3.2 cm for the combination group (25).

As encouraging as these results are, they reflect only the first year of data from the collaborative study. These patients clearly must be followed (the study is now in its third year) to document whether growth acceleration continues with all or any of the various treatment regimens. Furthermore, although no toxicity resulting from hGH therapy was evident, including effects on glucose tolerance, continued documentation of safety is required. Despite these caveats, the results of the first year of the study are highly encouraging and suggest that a satisfactory therapy for the short stature of Turner syndrome may now be available.

REFERENCES

1. Turner HH. A syndrome of infantilism, congenital webbed neck, and cubitus valgus. Endocrinology 23:566–574, 1938.

2. Palmer CG, Reichmann A. Chromosomal and clinical findings in 110 females with Turner syndrome. Hum. Genet. 35:35–49, 1976.

3. Park E, Bailey JD, Cowell CA. Growth and maturation of patients with Turner's syndrome. Pediatr. Res. 17:1–7, 1983.

4. Brook CGD, Murset G, Zachmann M, Prader A. Growth in children with 45,XO Turner's syndrome. Arch Dis. Child. 49:789–795, 1974.

5. Lev-Ran A. Androgens, estrogens, and the ultimate height in XO gonadal dysgenesis. Am. J. Dis. Child. 131:648–649, 1977.

6. Sybert VP. Adult height in Turner syndrome with and without androgen therapy. J. Pediatr. 104:365–369, 1984.

7. Ranke MB, Pfluger H, Rosendahl W, et al. Turner syndrome: Sponta-

neous growth in 150 cases and review of the literature. Eur. J. Pediatr. 141:81–88, 1983.

8. Brook CGD. Growth hormone deficiency in Turner's syndrome. N. Engl. J. Med. 298:1203–1204, 1978.

9. Faggiano M, Minozzi M, Lombardi G, Carella G, Criscuolo T. Two cases of the chromatin positive variety of ovarian dysgenesis (XO/XX mosaicism) associated with hGH deficiency and marginal impairment of other hypothalamic functions. Clin. Genet. 8:324–329, 1975.

10. Duke EMC, Hussein DH, Hamilton W. Turner's syndrome associated with growth hormone deficiency. Scott. Med. J. 26:240–244, 1981.

11. Laczi F, Julesz J, Janaky T, Laszlo FA. Growth hormone reserve capacity in Turner's syndrome. Horm. Metab. Res. 11:664–666, 1979.

12. Ross JL, Long LM, Loriaux DL, Cutler GB Jr. Growth hormone secretory dynamics in Turner syndrome. J. Pediatr. 106:202–206, 1985.

13. Cuttler L, Van Vliet G, Conte FA, Kaplan SA, Grumbach MM. Somatomedin-C levels in children and adolescents with gonadal dysgenesis: Differences from age-matched normal females and effect of chronic estrogen replacement therapy. J. Clin. Endocrinol. Metab. 60: 1087–1092, 1985.

14. Rosenfeld RG, Hintz RL, Johanson AJ, et al. Prospective, randomized trial of methionyl human growth hormone and/or oxandrolone in Turner syndrome. J. Pediatr. 109: 936–942, 1986.

15. Rosenfeld RG, Dollar LA, Hintz RL, Conover C. Normal somatomedin-C/insulin-like growth factor I binding and action in cultured human fibroblasts from Turner syndrome. Acta Endocrinol. (Copenh.) 104: 502–509, 1983.

16. Urban MD, Lee PA, Dorst JP, Plotnick LP, Migeon CJ. Oxandrolone therapy in patients with Turner syndrome. J. Pediatr. 94:823–827, 1979.

17. Lenko HL, Perheentupa J, Soderholm A. Growth in Turner's syndrome: Spontaneous and fluoxymesterone stimulated. Acta Pediatr. Scand. (Suppl.) 277:57–63, 1979.

18. Ross JL, Cassorla FG, Skerda MC, Valk IM, Loriaux DL, Cutler GB Jr. A preliminary study of the effect of estrogen dose on growth in Turner's syndrome. N. Engl. J. Med. 309:1104–1106, 1983.

19. Hutchings JJ, Escamilla RF, Li CH, Forsham PH. Li human growth hormone administration in gonadal dysgenesis. Am. J. Dis. Child. 109: 318–321, 1965.

20. Tzagournis M. Response to long-term administration of human growth hormone in Turner's syndrome. J. Am. Med. Assoc. 210:2373–2376, 1969.

21. Butenandt O. Growth hormone deficiency and growth hormone therapy in Ullrich-Turner Syndrome. Klin. Wochenschr. 58:99–101, 1980.

22. Stahnke N. Human growth hormone treatment in short children without growth hormone deficiency. N. Engl. J. Med. 310:925–926, 1984.

23. Rudman D, Goldsmith M, Kutner M, Blackston D. Effect of growth hormone and oxandrolone singly and together on growth rate in girls with X chromosome abnormalities. J. Pediatr. 96:132–135, 1980.

24. Ranke MB. Spontanes wachstum beim Turner-syndrom. Der Kinderarzt 9:1205–1208, 1985.

25. Bayley N, Pinneau SR. Tables for predicting adult height from skeletal age: Revised for use with the Greulich-Pyle hand standards. J. Pediatr. 40:423–441, 1952.

9

Growth Hormone as a Potential Adjunctive Therapy for Weight Loss

DAVID R. CLEMMONS
and LOUIS E. UNDERWOOD
University of North Carolina
School of Medicine
Chapel Hill, North Carolina

Growth hormone therapy for weight reduction has been advocated for several years (1). Its use was proposed after it was shown that injection of GH results in release of free fatty acids and glycerol into the blood of laboratory animals (2) and that these short-term responses could be maintained over long time periods (3). In addition, carcass analyses of rats (4) and pigs (5) confirmed that long-term injection of GH causes a reduction in total body fat content. Besides its lipolytic properties, treatment with GH causes significant nitrogen retention (6). As with lipolysis, nitrogen conservation persists during long-term GH therapy, and carcass analyses have shown increases in muscle mass (4,5). The rationale for using an anabolic agent in the therapy of obesity is based on the observation that prolonged fasting is accompanied by significant losses of total body nitrogen (7). As a result, weight loss in obese patients is accompanied by an obligatory loss of muscle mass. Although this reduction in muscle mass has not been proven to account for the weakness and easy fatigue that occur during long-term weight loss, it is possible that the two are related. Therefore, the rationale for giving GH to obese subjects engaged in dietary restriction is that it offers the potential to facilitate fat loss and nitrogen retention.

To establish the effectiveness of GH therapy in facilitating weight loss and protein sparing, an optimal diet must be ingested. This diet should permit maximal fat loss, maximal nitrogen sparing, and high compliance. The degree to which this can be achieved is limited by the apparent requirement of some nitrogen wasting to achieve fat loss. The diet also should be designed to optimize the anabolic and lipolytic response to GH therapy. Such stringent requirements mandate preliminary studies that test the efficacy of specific diets to achieve maximal nitrogen sparing and weight loss, prior to testing the combination of GH and diet therapy. During the past 3 years we have conducted a series of studies in normal weight and obese volunteers to assess the efficacy of test diets in achieving weight loss and in conserving nitrogen. We have measured nitrogen retention by classical balance study techniques and have determined the effect of dietary manipulations on plasma somatomedin C concentrations.

Somatomedin-C (insulinlike growth factor I, IGF-I) is a peptide growth factor whose plasma levels are under the control of both nutritional status and growth hormone. Somatomedin-C has been shown to stimulate protein synthesis in muscle (8) and its plasma concentrations may be closely linked to protein metabolism. Measurement of Sm-C offers the potential of a simple blood test that defines the interaction between GH therapy and nutritional status, because its fluctuations reflect the net effect of both.

I.   EFFECT OF FASTING ON PLASMA Sm- C/IFG-I AND NITROGEN BALANCE

In our first study we fasted seven obese male volunteers for 10 days. This total food deprivation resulted in a decrease in mean plasma Sm-C concentrations from 0.83 ± 0.26 (1 SD) U/ml to 0.21 ± 0.18 U/ml ($p < .001$). More importantly, this decline in plasma Sm-C

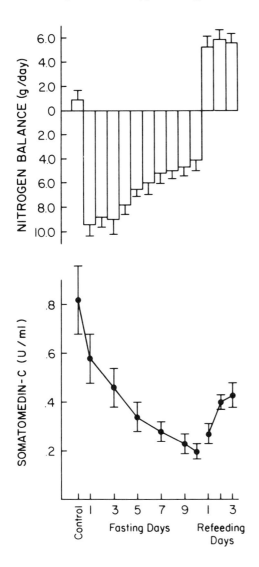

Figure 1. Changes in plasma Sm-C concentrations and in nitrogen balance during fasting. Seven slightly obese volunteers were fasted for 10 days, receiving water ad libitum, vitamins, and potassium chloride. (From Ref. 9.)

correlated with changes in nitrogen balance ($r = .74$) (9). These results indicated the immunoreactive Sm-C was under nutritional control, and since GH secretion was intact in these subjects, it suggested
that nutritional intake was at least as important as GH in controlling
plasma Sm-C concentrations.

II. DIETARY COMPOSITION THAT
REGULATES Sm-C/IGF-I IN PLASMA

To assess the dietary variables that controlled Sm-C concentrations,
and to determine if this test could be used to monitor the response
to diets of variable composition, five normal-weight volunteers were
fasted for three 5-day periods. Each fast was followed by a 5-day test
diet and a 2-week equilibration period on a control diet. Each subject
served as his or her own control. The test diets were of the following
composition: 1.) control protein 1.35 g/kg ideal body weight, control
calories 35.3 kcal/kg; 2.) control calories 35 kcal/kg, low protein 0.43
g/kg; 3.) low protein 0.40 g/kg, low energy 11 kcal/kg. All subjects
showed significant reductions (average decrease = 64%) in mean
plasma Sm-C levels during the 5-day fasting period. The subjects who
were refed the control diet had significant increases in plasma Sm-C
values from a nadir of 0.67 ± 0.15 U/ml to 1.26 ± 0.2 U/ml after 5
days ($p < .001$) (10). In contrast, subjects who were refed the low
protein, control energy diet showed increases to a mean value of 0.90
± 0.24 U/ml. This response was significantly less than the subjects
receiving the control diet ($p < .05$ compared to the response to the
control diet). The diet with deficient calories resulted in a further
reduction in plasma Sm-C to 0.31 ± 0.06 U/ml. This study also
showed that plasma Sm-C values reflect accurately the nitrogen balance response to the test diet. When the change in Sm-C concentration
during each fast and diet period was compared to the mean daily
nitrogen balance for each interval, the correlation was $r = .90$. It
appeared therefore that plasma Sm-C concentrations could be used to
monitor the effects of changes in dietary composition.

Because plasma Sm-C values continued to decline when subjects
received the 11 kcal/kg diet, we concluded that there is a minimum
caloric intake needed to permit a response in plasma Sm-C values. To
determine the level of caloric intake that would permit an increase in
Sm-C after a fasting-induced decrease, six volunteers were fasted for 5
days then refed three diets in succession, all containing optimal protein

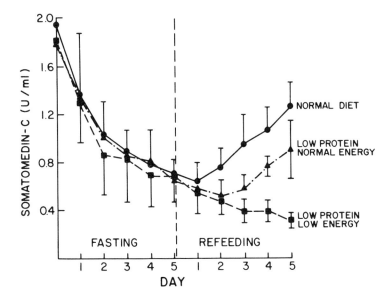

Figure 2. Changes in plasma Sm-C concentrations in five normal weight volunteers who were fasted for three occasions for five days then refed one of three diets. See text for composition of diets. (From Ref. 10.)

(1.0 g/kg) and three separate energy compositions (11, 18, or 25 kcal/kg). For comparison, the same subjects were restudied during ingestion of three diets containing optimal energy (35 kcal/kg) and three separate protein intakes (0.2, 0.4, and 1.0 g/kg). The results showed that despite normal protein intake, between 11 and 18 kcal/kg was required for any significant increase in plasma Sm-C to occur. This suggested that a minimal intake of energy is needed to conserve protein sufficient to permit any increase in the plasma concentration of this factor (11). Since the change in Sm-C correlated well with changes in nitrogen balance ($r = .88$) during this study, it appears that plasma Sm-C measurements may be helpful in deciding the absolute lower limit of caloric intake that can be used to treat obesity and still preserve protein.

Because protein appeared to be an important determinant of maximal restoration of Sm-C to control levels, we carried out a study designed to determine whether supplementation of the diet with essen-

tial amino acids would influence the rate of increases in the concentration of Sm-C after fasting (12). During two 5-day fasting periods,
plasma Sm-C concentrations fell 64% from control levels of 1.64 ±
0.24 and 1.61 ± 0.21 U/ml to 0.67 ± 0.18 and 0.74 ± 0.17 U/ml,
respectively ($p < .001$). Following ingestion of a diet that was supplemented with essential amino acids (EAA) (e.g., 80% of total nitrogen
supplied as EAA), the Sm-C values rose to 1.41 ± 0.19 U/ml, and this
value was significantly greater than if a nonsupplemented (20% of total
nitrogen supplied as EAA) diet was ingested (1.15 ± 0.15 U/ml; $p <$
.02). Here also, changes in nitrogen balance correlated with these
responses ($r = .81$). From these studies it appeared that the ratio of
essential amino acids to total nitrogen in the diet also controls the

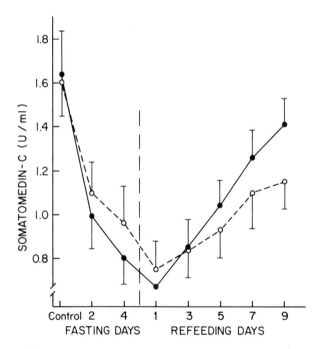

Figure 3. Changes in plasma Sm-C concentrations in healthy volunteers
who were fasted on two separate occasions for five days, then refed diets
either supplemented with essential amino acids (solid line) or not supplemented (dashed line). Composition of refeeding diets given in text. (From
Ref. 12.)

degree of protein preservation and the plasma Sm-C response that can be achieved.

To determine if changes observed with these fasting/refeeding models were applicable to the dietary treatment of obese subjects, six obese (two males, four females) volunteers who were between 30 and 70% over ideal body weight were studied for two 3-week intervals during which they received two test diets. These diets were not preceded by fasting but were preceded by a 1-week equilibration period in which a 35 kcal/kg diet was ingested. Both test diets contained 12 kcal/kg, and one included protein supplementation such that each subject ingested 1.0 g protein/kg. The other diet contained 15% of calories as protein, or approximately 0.34 g/kg. During ingestion of the supplemented diet, nitrogen balance was significantly less negative (-3.34 ± 0.56 g/day) and a mean weight loss of 3.88 ± 1.37 kg. The nonsupplemented diet resulted in significantly more negative balance (-5.40 ± 0.98; $p < .01$) and a total weight loss of 4.09 ± 0.83 kg (not significant, NS). Changes in plasma Sm-C values reflected these changes in protein metabolism, decreasing from a baseline of 1.27 ± 0.74 U/ml to 0.63 ± 0.27 U/ml on the nonsupplemented diet, and to 0.79 ± 0.42 U/ml on the protein-supplemented diet. Comparison of the mean absolute Sm-C values showed that there were significant differences on days 8, 12, and 14 of the test diets. The change in plasma Sm-C, therefore, reflected the protein-sparing effects of the higher protein diet. It appears that measurement of plasma Sm-C can be used to design diets for the therapy of obesity that result in maximal protein sparing while trying to achieve optimal weight loss.

III. USE OF GH AS AN ADJUNCT TO WEIGHT REDUCTION

Even optimal diet weight-reduction therapy, however, results in slow rates of weight loss, and the diets that increase protein retention do not accelerate lipolysis. Similarly, agents that accelerate lipolysis, such as thyroxine, also accelerate protein breakdown. Growth hormone may obviate some of these shortcomings. Chung et al. treated 11 young swine with 22 µg/kg/day porcine growth hormone for 12 weeks (5). These animals were permitted to ingest food ad libitum. The growth hormone–treated animals gained significantly more weight (19.8 vs. 17.5 kg; $p < .01$) than control animals and had no difference in adipose content of the carcass while gaining significantly greater muscle mass (24.0 vs. 21.1 kg; $p < .05$). In these young growing animals, therefore, GH therapy caused a redistribution of weight to the muscle compartment at the expense of the fat compartment. One possible reason that there was no decrease in fat content is that unrestricted food intake was permitted.

Because of limited availability of hGH prior to production by recombinant DNA techniques, only a few studies of dietary manipulation have been performed with this agent. Bray fed eight obese adult volunteers a diet containing 450 calories for 11–16 days, then administered 8 mg GH daily for 4 days (13). He noted that the oxygen consumption was increased from a mean of 21.8 L/min to 24.5 L/min ($p < .01$) on GH therapy. Therefore, the effect of GH could be detected despite 11–16 days of feeding a severely restricted diet (13). In a follow-up study, Bray et al. showed that obese volunteers being fed 900 cal/day and receiving triiodothyronine (T_3) were in significant negative nitrogen balance (14). Treatment with 5 mg GH daily for 14 days resulted in enhancement of oxygen consumption in four subjects and nitrogen retention. Two subjects did not respond to GH with improved nitrogen retention. Schwarz et al. starved three obese volunteers for 12 days, while administering GH every other day (15). Growth hormone injections improved nitrogen balance compared to a control interval, with mean nitrogen loss being -3.5 g/day on GH compared to -6.2 g/day during the control period. Similarly, free fatty acid levels were higher on the days that the subjects received GH. Felig and co-workers fasted five obese subjects for 31 days then administered 5 mg GH daily for 3 days and compared this to their response in the fed state (16). The effect of GH on nitrogen balance was difficult to interpret, because while there was significant retention of urinary urea nitrogen excretion, ammonia excretion increased. As a result, total urinary nitrogen remained unchanged, suggesting that protein was not preserved.

Because of these studies and the recent availability of biosynthetic hGH, we have carried out a pilot study attempting to determine the short-term efficacy of GH therapy as an adjunct to diet therapy for obesity. Eight obese volunteers who were 23–67% over ideal body weight were fed a modestly restricted diet containing 24 kcal/kg and 1.0 g protein/kg for 11 weeks. Growth hormone (0.1 mg/kg ideal body weight) was injected intramuscularly every other day for 3 weeks.

Saline injections were also given for a 3-week interval, and the order of these treatments was randomized. While the subjects were receiving GH, nitrogen balance was significantly improved. Nitrogen losses were 0.35 ± 2.14 g/day on GH, compared to -2.21 ± 1.45 g/day on vehicle alone ($p < .001$). Using Reifenstein's formula to estimate loss of lean body mass, GH therapy resulted in a loss of 0.2 kg compared to 1.25 kg with saline injections ($p < .01$). The differences in total weight loss and loss of adipose tissue were not significant. However, there were significant individual variations in fat loss. Of the six subjects who had usable measurements three had fat losses of 3.1, 3.12, 2.5 kg while receiving GH, compared to 0.82, 2.2, and 0.81 kg respectively on vehicle alone. The other subjects, however, showed no preferential fat loss. The mean fat losses were 3.06 ± 1.39 kg with GH compared to 2.64 ± 1.08 kg with vehicle (NS). Plasma Sm-C concentrations increased substantially in all subjects, rising from a mean of 0.86 ± 0.28 U/ml (control) to a peak value of 3.20 ± 1.6 U/ml on day 12 of GH therapy. Somatomedin-C values did not change significantly when vehicle alone was injected, indicating that the modest caloric restriction was not sufficient to lower Sm-C values in these subjects. The degree of increase in Sm-C was surprising in view of the fact that the subjects were catabolic. It indicates that this measurement is a very sensitive index of GH status, and that further caloric restriction may be possible without impairing the anabolic response to GH.

The subjects in this study had minimal side effects. Most had minor fluid retention during GH therapy. This was followed by a diuresis when therapy was completed. Glucose tolerance was stable in all subjects. Mean fasting glucose on vehicle injection was 92.8 ± 10.0 mg/dl and was 96.0 ± 16.0 mg/dl (NS) on GH therapy. Similarly, fasting insulin levels showed no increase during GH therapy.

We conclude from these studies that injections of GH to obese subjects who are ingesting a calorically restricted diet results in nitrogen sparing and does not retard weight loss. Whether GH therapy results in accelerated fat loss is uncertain and requires further study. It is possible that GH will increase the rate of lipolysis in selected subjects but will not be effective uniformly. It is also possible that improved measurements of body fat content such as nuclear magnetic resonance will lead to more accurate estimates of fat loss. Finally, since GH responsiveness was preserved on 24 kcal/kg, it is possible that more severe caloric restriction will permit an improved lipolytic response without impairing the anabolic response to GH therapy.

REFERENCES

1. Bray GA, Davidson MG, Drenick EJ. Obesity: A serious symptom. Ann. Inter. Med. 77:797–805, 1972.

2. Knobil E. Direct evidence for fatty acid mobilization in response to growth hormone administration in rat. Proc. Soc. Exp. Biol. Med. 101:288–289, 1959.

3. Raben MS, Hollenberg CH. Effect of growth hormone on plasma free fatty acids. J. Clin. Invest. 38:484–490, 1959.

4. Greenbaum AL. Changes in body composition and respiratory quotient of normal fed rats treated with purified growth hormone. Biochem. J. 54:400–407, 1953.

5. Chung CS, Etherton TD, Wiggins JP. Stimulation of swine growth by porcine growth hormone. J. Animal Sci. 60:118–130, 1985.

6. Russell JA. Effects of growth hormone on protein and carbohydrate metabolism. Am. J. Clin. Nutr. 5:404–409, 1957.

7. Owen OE, Felig P, Morgan AP, Wahren J, Cahill GF Jr. Liver and kidney metabolism in prolonged starvation. J. Clin. Invest. 48:1589–1596, 1967.

8. Salmon WD Jr, DuVall MR. In vitro stimulation of leucine incorporation into muscle and cartilage protein by a serum fraction with sulfation factor activity differentiation of effects from those of growth hormone and insulin. Endocrinology 87:1168–1180, 1970.

9. Clemmons DR, Klibanski A, Underwood LR, Ridgway EC, MacArthur JW, Bietens IZ, Van Wyk JJ. Reduction in plasma immunoreactive somatomedin-C during fasting in humans. J. Clin. Endocrinol. Metab. 53:1247–1250, 1981.

10. Isley WL, Underwood LE, Clemmons DR. Dietary components that regulate serum somatomedin-C concentrations in humans. J. Clin. Invest. 71:175–182, 1983.

11. Isley WL, Underwood LE, Clemmons DR. Changes in plasma somatomedin-C in response to ingestion of diets with variable protein and energy content. J. Parenteral and Enteral Nutr. 8:364–369, 1984.

12. Clemmons DR, Seek MM, Underwood LE. Supplemental essential amino acids augment the somatomedin-C/IGF-I response to refeeding after fasting. Metabolism 34:391–395, 1985.

13. Bray GA. Calorigenic effect of human growth hormone in obesity. J. Clin. Endocrinol. Metab. 29:119–122, 1969.

14. Bray GA, Raben MS, Londono J, Gallagher TF Jr. Effects of tri-iodothyronine, growth hormone and anabolic steroids on nitrogen excretion and oxygen consumption of obese patients. J. Clin. Endocrinol. Metab. 33:293–300, 1971.

15. Schwarz, F, der Kinderen PJ, van Riet HG, Thijssen JHH, van Wayjen RGA. Influence of exogenous growth hormone on the metabolism of fasting obese patients. Metabolism 21:297–303, 1972.

16. Felig P, Marliss EB, Cahill GF Jr. Metabolic response to human growth hormone during prolonged starvation. J. Clin. Invest. 50:411–421, 1971.

10

Growth Hormone, the Somatomedins, and Aging

RAYMOND L. HINTZ

Stanford University School of Medicine
Stanford, California

I. THE GROWTH HORMONE–SOMATOMEDIN–GROWTH HORMONE-RELEASING FACTOR/SOMATOSTATIN SYSTEM

Over the past three decades it has become clear that much of the control of somatic growth is by way of pituitary growth hormone and the growth factors under the control of growth hormone. Many of the biological actions of GH are mediated through the somatomedins (1). There are two somatomedins known to circulate in human plasma:

Supported in part by grants AG 01213 and AM 24085 from the National Institutes of Health.

Insulinlike growth factor I (IGF-I), also known as somatomedin C (Sm-C), is a 70 amino acid peptide with approximately 50% homology to human proinsulin (2,3). Insulinlike growth factor II (IGF-II) circulates in plasma and has approximately 80% homology to IGF-I and nearly 50% homology to human proinsulin (4). Both of these growth factors are under GH control, although it is clear that IGF-I/Sm-C is more tightly under GH control than IGF-II. Insulinlike growth factor II attains maximal levels with a relatively small amount of GH secretion. Separate receptor sites for the insulinlike growth factors have been found. Sm-C/IGF-I receptor sites seem to be ubiquitous through all cell types that have been examined, and in many cases these receptor sites have been shown to be linked to cell action. Specific receptor sites for IGF-II appear to be less widely distributed and are less clearly linked to biological action.

The original "somatomedin hypothesis" held that essentially all the biological actions of GH were mediated through the somatomedins (5). It is now clear that there are certain direct actions of GHs that are not mediated by the somatomedins. However, compelling evidence has been developed that somatomedins can cause growth in vivo in the absence of GH. Schoenle and Froesch demonstrated that the in vivo growth-promoting action of pure IGF-I and IGF-II can essentially duplicate GH action (6). These data strengthen the potential role of the somatomedin peptides as the major mediator of GH effects on growth and anabolism. However, it is likely that this hypothesis is too simple. The work of Stiles et al. (7), as well as our own work (8), suggests that peptides act on many cell types in concert and in synergism with other growth factors and hormones from plasma or tissues.

Growth hormone, like other anterior pituitary hormones, is under the control of hypothalamic neuropeptides secreted into the hypophyseal–portal system. Somatostatin (SRIF) was originally isolated as a potent inhibitor of GH secretion from the pituitary gland (9). It is also widespread in other tissues and plays a variety of metabolic roles. For a long time there has been good biological evidence that a simulator (growth hormone releasing factor, GRF) must also exist. Attempts to isolate the GRF from hypothalamic tissues directly were unsuccessful, but it was isolated and sequenced from tumor tissue (10). Growth hormone releasing factor is a potent stimulator of GH release and secretion, and it appears to be limited in its distribution to the hypothalamus. The somatomedins also play a role in the control of GH secretion. Berelowitz et al. showed that Sm-C/IGF-I stimulated the production of somatostatin by hypothalamic tissues, thus having a net inhibitory effect on GH secretion (11). It has also been shown that the somatomedins have a direct action on the pituitary glands in vitro to block the action of GH-releasing factor, thereby inhibiting GH secretion. Thus the somatomedins inhibit the secretion of GH in at least two ways, and the GH-SM-GRF/SRIF system is organized in a classic feedback loop structure.

II. METABOLISM AND AGING

Aging is a complex phenomenon that has many metabolic consequences, among them a loss of regenerative capacity of tissues (12), a decrease of protein synthesis with a net loss of body protein (13), and a decrease in bone mass (14). The complications of aging can be viewed to a large extent as being the result of the inability to adequately replace cell and protein losses. Growth hormone and growth factors are major regulators of cell division and protein synthesis. Among the peptide growth factors that have been purified and shown to be powerful stimulants of cell growth in vitro are the nerve growth factors (15), epidermal growth factor (16), fibroblast growth factor (17), myoblast growth factor (18), and thymosin (19), as well the somatomedins or insulinlike growth factors (20). All of them share the ability to evoke in cells a series of events leading to cell division that has been characterized as the "positive pleiotypic response" (21). Most of these growth factors seem to be tissue specific in their actions, as is suggested by their names. However, the somatomedin or insulinlike growth factor peptides have very broad tissue specificity compared to the other growth factors.

Since many of the complications of aging can be viewed as the result of the inability to adequately replace cell and protein losses, it is important for researchers interested in the aging process to study changes in the secretion and action of the major anabolic hormones during aging. Studies of growth hormone and growth hormone action in aging indicate that there are major alterations not only in levels of GH and Sm-C/IGF-I, but also in the control of GH secretion at the hypothalamic level. In every case, the changes observed fit the overall hypothesis that changes in the growth hormone–somatomedin system are responsible for at least part of the lack of anabolic action in aging, and therefore may play a role in the development of the complications of the aging process.

III. GROWTH HORMONE, SOMATOMEDIN, AND AGING

Differences in GH secretion between aging individuals and normal controls were first proposed in the 1960s (22,23). Bazzarre and co-workers, using both stimulated secretion of GH and integrated 24-hour GH concentrations, found that GH secretion decreased with age, particularly after the age of 50 (24). Later studies have not only confirmed the decrease in GH but linked it to a decline in Sm-C/IGF-I. The studies of Rudman and his group also found a link between Sm-C/IGF-I and body-to-mass ratio in aging (25). In collaboration with Florini, Prinz, and Vitiello (26), we looked at the relationship among Sm-C/IGF-I, aging, and GH secretion rates. We were able to show that there is a highly significant negative correlation between age and Sm-C/IGF-I concentrations in men above 40 years old. Thus as men age, the plasma concentration of Sm-C/IGF-I, a major anabolic hormone, also decreases. Furthermore, in an intensively studied subset of these patients we were able to show a correlation between GH secretion and Sm-C/IGF-I concentrations ($r = .598$, $p < .034$). The most likely interpretation of the data is that GH secretion decreases with aging, and the level of the GH-dependent growth factor Sm-C/IGF-I decreases commensurately. The studies of Sm-C/IGF-I concentrations in aging are summarized in Table 1.

The negative correlation between Sm-C/IGF-I levels and age has been shown in females as well as males. In a study of more than 80

Table 1. Sm-C/IGF-I Levels in Aging

Study	Percentage of young adult control	Sex
Bazzarre (24)	38	Male
Rudman (25)	27	Male
Florini (26)	72	Male
Bennett (27)	65	Female

aging women, we observed that Sm-C/IGF-I concentrations decreased with age ($r = -.47$, $p < .001$). In contrast, the level of the other human somatomedin peptide, IGF-II, does not decrease with age. There was no relationship shown between Sm-C/IGF-I levels and accelerated osteoporosis in these women, but the covariation among age, Sm-C/IGF-I, and senile osteoporosis does not rule out such a relationship (27).

A crucial unanswered question is whether the low levels of GH and Sm-C/IGF-I have any biological relevance. We are now in the midst of a study of GH, Sm-C/IGF-I, and muscle strength as estimated by grip strength in a population of aging men and women. Thus far ($n = 31$) the results show that Sm-C/IGF-I is significantly correlated with both age ($r = -.518$, $p < .001$) and grip strength ($r = -.474$, $p < .01$). Although these observations do not prove causation, they do provide support for the hypothesis that some of the catabolic changes of aging, could be linked to the decrease in growth factors such as Sm-C/IGF-I.

The decline in GH secretion rates with age could be caused by a decrease in growth hormone releasing factor (GRF) secretion, an increase in somatostatin tone, or secretory failure by the pituitary cell. Thus far it is unclear which one of these accounts for the decrease in GH secretion. In several studies of normal adult volunteers, most individuals over the age of 50 fail to respond to bolus injection of GRF. However, this could result from an increase of somatostatin tone, which effectively blocks reaction to GRF, or to failure of pituitary GH secretion. Further studies will be necessary to unravel the possible explanations.

IV. RESPONSE TO SHORT-TERM GROWTH HORMONE TREATMENT

In contrast to the brisk anabolic response of children and adults with growth hormone deficiency to growth hormone, relatively small doses of growth hormone (0.168 U per kilogram body weight to the ¾ power daily) produced little biological effect in normal adult volunteers (28). In contrast, our studies in normal adult volunteers with the biosynthetic methionyl GH (29) showed impressive biological effects to short-term GH administration. The major difference between these two studies was dosage. An average dose given to adults in the earlier studies was approximately 2 mg/day, whereas the biosynthetic studies were done with 8 mg/day. The failure to show clear biological effects in the studies with low GH doses may be due to the suppression of GH secretion by exogenous GH, so that the total amount of GH available to the subject was unchanged when the normal individuals were treated.

Although the cause of the decline in GH secretion with age is at present unknown, this observation does lead to the hope that the low Sm-C/IGF-I concentration and perhaps some of the lack of anabolism in aging could be corrected by exogenous GH therapy. In studies comparing the biological response to GH of aging men, hypopituitary adults, and normal adults, Bazzarre and co-workers showed that the response of the aging men was similar to that of hypopituitary adults at low (1.0 mg daily) dosages of GH (24). Furthermore, Johanson and Blizzard showed that treatment of aging individuals with these dosages of GH was also associated with a rise of plasma Sm-C/IGF-I concentrations (30). However, no short-term studies have been done comparing aging individuals to normal controls at higher dosage of growth hormone, and no long-term studies of GH action on aging have yet been published.

V. IN VITRO SOMATOMEDIN ACTION IN AGING

In addition to the age-associated changes in GH secretion and somatomedin peptide levels, there are also changes at the end organ level. For the past several years we have studied human fibroblasts in culture as an in vitro model for somatomedin action. Much of the previous work on aging in vitro was done on transformed and/or nonhuman cells. We feel that the nontransformed human fibroblast system is more likely to give answers of physiological relevance. In this cell culture system we can determine Sm-C/IGF-I receptor sites as well as IGF-II receptor sites (31). Insulinlike growth factor II receptors are more plentiful on the surface of these normal human fibroblasts than either Sm-C/IGF-I or insulin receptors. We have also determined the biological effects of growth factors and hormones on normal fibroblasts in culture (8). In these normal fibroblast cultures, Sm-C/IGF-I stimulates both cell division and protein synthesis, consistent with the apparent affinity of the receptor site. In contrast, no direct actions of GH have been seen in this system. The effect of IGF-I is potentiated by low (0.25%) concentrations of hypopituitary human serum, suggesting that cofactors are important in SM/IGF action. This low concentration of human hypopituitary serum can be at least partially replaced by FGF or EGF. When the cells are preincubated with dexamethasone (0.1 μM), the effect is synergistic. In fact, the combination of SM/IGF, dexamethasone, and 0.25% HHS is equal to or better than the effect of 20% fetal calf serum on cell division. This synergistic effect of dexamethasone is seen only on cell division and not on protein synthesis or amino acid transport.

Our studies show that fibroblasts from all age groups are dependent on Sm-C/IGF-I for stimulation of cell multiplication as well as such metabolic functions as protein and RNA synthesis. Dexamethasone has no direct effect on cell multiplication at any age but acts synergistically with Sm-C/IGF-I to cause an increase in ^{3}H-thymidine incorporation and cell number in cells from children or adults. Early passage fibroblast cultures from aging patients have the same generation time, Sm-C/IGF-I receptor affinity and number per cell,

Table 2.   Effect of Aging on Fibroblast Response

Donor age (years)	SM	SM + HHS	SM + HHS + DEX
7–24	8.1	26.4	47.3
60–96	7.8	20.3	17.9

Results expressed as fold increase in ³H-thymidine uptake over baseline. Recalculation of data in Refs. 32 and 33. Means of 10 to 15 experiments. SM = Sm-C, 50 ng/ml; HHS = human hypopituitary serum, 0.25%; DEX = dexamethasone, 0.1 m*M*.

and response to pure Sm-C/IGF-I as do cells from adults under 40 years old (32). However, fibroblast cultures from aging individuals show a marked difference in their response to dexamethasone pretreatment. In the presence of dexamethasone the cells fail to show the synergistic response expected but actually show a decrease in the ability to respond to IGF. This appears to be due mainly to a shift in the time course of thymidine biosynthesis. This failure to show synergism to dexamethasone is reflected not only in DNA synthesis studies but also in cell division studies. The combination of dexamethasone, hypopituitary serum, and maximal amounts of Sm-C/IGF-I is unable to induce cells from aging individuals to divide as rapidly as cells from normal individuals (33). These results are summarized in Table 2. The human fibroblast system provides a model which will allow the dissection of the effects of other hormones and factors on the action of IGF on human cells and the changes caused by the aging process.

VI.   SUMMARY AND CONCLUSION

Many of the complications of aging can be viewed as consequences of decreased anabolism and tissue renewal. Since growth hormone and the somatomedin peptides have been shown to be major components of anabolism, they are logical targets for study in aging. Not only is there a decrease in GH secretion with aging, but this decrease in GH secretion is reflected in lower Sm-C/IGF-I concentrations in blood. Thus many aging individuals appear to be functionally hypopituitary. In addition, there are abnormalities in the hypothalamic peptides controlling GH which need further delineation. This functional GH deficiency of the aging could play a role in the catabolic complications of aging.

The preliminary studies of GH treatment of aging individuals show that low doses of GH produce short-term metabolic responses and Sm-C/IGF-I responses comparable to those observed in GH-treated hypopituitary individuals. However, long-term studies have not yet been done to determine whether the treatment of aging individuals with exogenous GH will slow or reverse any component of the aging process. In addition to the evidence for functional hypopituitarism of aging, our data on Sm-C/IGF-I action in the human fibroblast model suggest that there is also a component of tissue resistance to Sm-C/IGF-I action which may limit or eliminate the ability of aging tissues to respond to the anabolic effects of GH. Only carefully done clinical studies will show whether GH has a therapeutic role in geriatric medicine.

REFERENCES

1. Hintz RL. Adv. Pediatr. 28:293, 1980.

2. Rinderknecht E, Humbel RE. J. Biol. Chem. 253:2769, 1978.

3. Svoboda ME, Van Wyk JJ, Klapper DG, et al. Biochemistry 19:790, 1980.

4. Rinderknecht E, Humbel RE. FEBS Lett. 89:283, 1978.

5. Daughaday WH, Hall K, Raben MS, et al. Nature 235:107, 1972.

6. Schoenle E, Froesch ER. Nature 296:252, 1982.

7. Stiles CD, Capone GT, Scher CD, et al. Proc. Natl. Acad. Sci. USA 76:1279, 1979.

8. Conover CA, Dollar LA, Hintz RL, Rosenfeld RG. J. Cell. Physiol. 116:191, 1983.

9. Brazeau P, et al. Science 179:77, 1973.

10. Guilleman R, et al. Science 218:585, 1982.

11. Berelowitz M, et al. Science 212:1279–1281, 1981.

12. Comfort A. The Biology of Senescence. Churchill Livingstone, London, 1979.

13. Winterer JC, Steffee WP, Davy W, et al. Exp. Gerontol. 11:79–87, 1976.

14. Smith RW. Fed. Proc. 6:1737, 1967.

15. Levi-Montalcini R. Ann. NY Acad. Sci. 118:149, 1964.

16. Cohn S. J. Biol. Chem. 237:1555, 1962.

17. Gospodarowicz D. Nature 249:123, 1974.

18. Gospodarowicz D, Wesesman J, Moran J. Nature 256:216, 1975.

19. White A, Goldstein AL. Adv. Metab. Disorders 8:259–374, 1975.

20. Van Wyk JJ, Underwood LE, Hintz RL, et al. Rec. Prog. Horm. Res. 30:259, 1974.

21. Hershko A, Mamont P, Shields R, et al. Nature (New Biol.) 232:206, 1971.

22. Finklestein J, Roffwarg H, Boyar R, et al. J. Clin. Endocrinol. Metab. 35:665, 1972.

23. Thompson R, Rodriguez A, Kowarski A, et al. J. Clin. Endocrinol. Metab. 35:334, 1972.

24. Bazzarre TL, Johanson AJ, Huseman CA, et al. In Growth Hormone and Related Peptides, Pecile A, Muller EE, eds., Excerpta Medica, Amsterdam, 1976, pp. 261–270.

25. Rudman D, et al. J. Clin. Invest. 67:1361, 1981.

26. Florini JR, Printz PN, Vitiello BS, Hintz RL. J. Gerontol. 40:2, 1985.

27. Bennett A, Wahner HW, Riggs BL, Hintz RL. J. Clin. Endocrinol. Metab. 59:701, 1985.

28. Rudman D, Chyatte S, Patterson J. J. Clin. Invest. 51:1941, 1975.

29. Hintz RL, et al. Lancet 1:1276, 1982.

30. Johanson AJ, Blizzard RM. Johns Hopkins Med. J. 149:115, 1981.

31. Thorsson AV, et al. J. Clin. Endocrinol. Metab. 60:387, 1985.

32. Conover CA, et al. J. Clin. Endocrinol. Metab. 60:685, 1985.

33. Conover CA, Rosenfeld RG, Hintz RL. J. Clin. Endocrinol. Metab. 61:423, 1985.

11

Pilot Studies Evaluating the Role of Growth Hormone in the Aging Process

ROBERT M. BLIZZARD, GARY BALIAN,
DOUGLAS L. NELSON,* JOHN SAVORY,
and ELIZABETH SUTPHEN†

University of Virginia
School of Medicine
Charlottesville, Virginia

STANTON H. COHN‡

Brookhaven National Laboratories
Upton, New York

ASHOK N. VASWANI
and JOHN F. ALOIA

Winthrop-University Hospital
Mineola, New York

ANN J. JOHANSON

Genentech, Inc.
South San Francisco, California

These studies were designed to consider two concepts. The first is that aging is related to diminished GH secretion; the second, that administration of GH will reverse or retard certain aspects of the aging process.

Current affiliations:
*Private practice, Newport News, Virginia.
†U.S. Army Foreign Science and Technology Center, Charlottesville, Virginia.
‡Stanford University School of Medicine, Stanford, California.

This work was supported by U.S.P.H.S. grants RR00948 and AG04303.

There were three objectives to be pursued: 1.) to determine if GH deficiency occurs with increasing age; 2.) to determine the acute metabolic response of normal elderly males to short-term (6 days) injections of GH; and 3.) to determine the long-term effect of GH over 3 years or more on the body composition of older men.

The data on the long-term effect of GH therapy are incomplete because this portion of the study was terminated when three GH-deficient patients who had received pituitary GH developed Creutzfeldt-Jakob disease. However, results in this pilot study are reported because the data may be useful for others who contemplate similar projects.

I. STUDY DESIGN

To determine whether GH deficiency occurs with aging, we measured plasma concentration of insulinlike growth factor I or somatomedin C (Sm-C) at various ages in adult males and females, and assessed GH secretion in eight males over 45 years of age by measuring blood GH concentrations every 20 minutes over a 24-hour period.

To determine acute metabolic response in normal elderly males to short-term (6 days) injection of GH, we placed five males over the age of 50 on constant diets for 2 weeks, collected daily 24-hour urine specimens for nitrogen and calcium, and measured plasma Sm-C concentrations. From day 8 to 14 the subjects received GH provided by the National Pituitary Hormone Distribution Program at a dosage of 3.5 IU/day.

To assess the long-term effect of GH treatment on body composition in the same five older men, GH was given each day initially, and when the Sm-C concentration reached the physiological range of young adults, the required dose (3.3 IU) was continued every other day. The intent had been to continue for at least 3 years, but these five subjects received GH for 8, 16, 22 (two subjects), and 24 months. The effect of GH on total body calcium, potassium, nitrogen, water, and bone density was determined before and after treatment. In addition, changes in composition of skin taken by biopsy from buttock areas were evaluated by electron microscopy, by determination of total collagen type by SDS-PAGE electrophoresis, and by determination of amino acid composition utilizing a Beckman 119 amino acid analyzer.

II. METHODS

Plasma somatomedin C concentrations were measured by Nichols Institute (1,2). All of the determinations for each sex were performed in two assays to minimize interassay variability. None of the 120 normal male and 96 normal female subjects were taking any medications, including birth control pills. Growth hormone was measured by a standard double antibody assay with a sensitivity of 0.5 ng/ml. All specimens from each individual were measured in one assay. Twenty microliters from each specimen from each patient were pooled and an integrated GH determination was done. Peaks of GH secretion were considered to be present if there were at least two consecutive determinations with at least one value above 2 ng/ml and the other above 1 ng/ml. Somatomedin C concentrations were measured several times before, during, and after the administration of GH. Urinary nitrogen and calcium were measured in each 24-hour urine using atomic absorption techniques. Total body calcium was measured at Brookhaven Laboratories by neutron activation (3), total body potassium by measuring naturally occurring potassium 40 (4), total body nitrogen by prompt neutron activation (5), total body water by tritium-labeled isotopic dilution techniques (6), and bone density by dual photon absorption techniques (7). The methods for measuring skin collagen structure and amino acid content have been reported elsewhere (8–10).

III. RESULTS

Among the females there is no apparent decline in Sm-C with age (Figure 1A). There is a significant decline, however, in the Sm-C concentrations in males between 23 and 45 years of age (Figure 1B). No further change was observed after the age of 45 years. The mean concentration for 55 females between 23 and 45 years was 0.66 U/ml ± 0.04 (SEM) and for 74 males between 23 and 45 it was 0.59 U/ml ± 0.04. For 41 females 46–77 years old, the mean concentration was 0.70 U/ml ± 0.59 U/ml ± 0.04, and for 46 males between 46 and 77 it was 0.42 U/ml ± 0.03.

The integrated concentrations of GH in the 8 males over 45 years of age were very low (0.6–1.1 ng/ml). Only one subject had more than

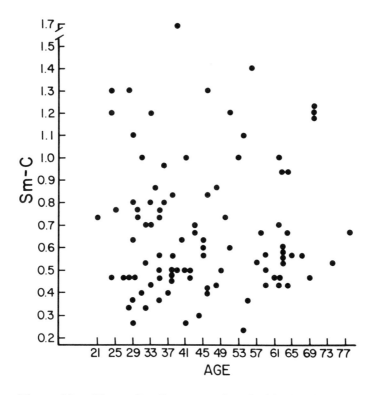

Figure 1A. Plasma Sm-C concentrations in 96 adult females who were in good health and not receiving any medications, including contraceptive pills. No decline of Sm-C with age was noted.

three peaks during a 24-hour period, and there were only 11 peaks of values greater than 4 ng/ml.

The acute effect of GH administration on nitrogen and calcium excretion is presented in Table 1. All five men excreted significantly less nitrogen when GH was given compared to the control period. An increased excretion of calcium during GH treatment was observed. These results are comparable to the effects we observed in GH-deficient children receiving GH. Simultaneously Sm-C determinations rose from a mean of 0.39 U/ml ± 0.01 SEM to 0.97 U/ml ± 0.01.

With GH therapy for 6–24 months, the Sm-C concentrations rose

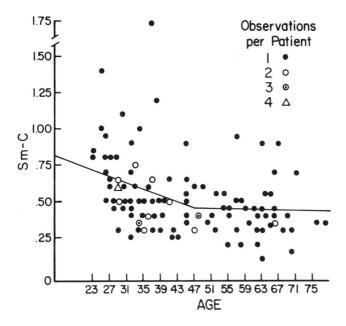

Figure 1B. Plasma Sm-C concentrations in 120 adult males who were in good health and not receiving any medications. A decline of Sm-C with age was noted for the individuals 23–45 years of age. After 45 years of age, no further change was observed.

Table 1. The Effect of GH Administration on Urinary Output of N^2 and Ca^{2+}

| Patient | Age (years) | Urinary | |
		N^{2a}	Ca^{2+b}
1 (RMB)	57	−0.85	+24.4
2 (JG)	54	−3.40	+48.1
3 (JH)	60	−3.38	+24.0
4 (MS)	64	−1.80	+11.9
5 (FM)	54	−2.32	+52.0

[a]Gm/24 hr; reflects positive N^2 balance.
[b]Mg/24 hr.

significantly (Figure 2), and body composition changed (Table 2). Subjects 2, 3, and 4 had what appeared to be significant increases in body weight, water, nitrogen, and phosphorus. In these three, the changes were consistent with an increase in muscle mass. Subjects 1 and 5 had no or only minimal changes in body nitrogen, potassium, phosphorus, and body water. Unfortunately, the changes of body composition observed in two of the controls (1 and 2) prevents our concluding that an increase in nitrogen truly occurred in subjects 2, 3, and 4 of the treatment group. Increase in body calcium of 4% or more

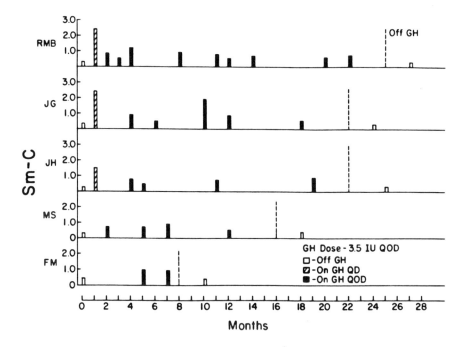

Figure 2. Plasma Sm-C changes with GH injection. Initially the Sm-C concentrations were in the very low range characteristically found in GH-deficient subjects. With GH injections the Sm-C rose significantly. The dosage was changed from 3.5 IU every day to 3.5 IU every other day to bring the Sm-C concentration into the range of 0.8–2.0 U. The dashed lines represent discontinuation of GH injections.

Table 2. Change in Body Composition with GH Administration

Subjects	Body weight (mo)			Body water (mo)			Body nitrogen (mo)			Body potassium (mo)			Body phosphorus (mo)			Body calcium (mo)		
	6	12	22	6	12	22	6	12	22	6	12	22	6	12	22	6	12	22
With GH therapy																		
Patient 1		+1.7%	+1.7%		−0.5%	−0.9%		−2%	−12%		−2.5%	−5.0%		0%	−4.8%		+4%	+4%
Patient 2		+3.3%	0%		+6.6%	+6.2%		+7%	+11%		+7.0%	+10.7%		+20%	+29%		+1.7%	−1.2%
Patient 3		+3.0%			+7.5%			+9%			+3%			+15%			0%	
Patient 4		+7.0%			+9.4%			+4%			+5.4%			+5%			+6%	
Patient 5	0%				+1.0%		+3%			+2%						+5%		
No GH therapy[a]																		
Control 1		+0.5%			0%			+5%			+2.5%			+1.9%			−0.5%	
Control 2		−7.7%			+0.5%			+7%			−5.3%			−7.7%			+0.8%	
Control 3		−3.3%			+0.9%			−11%			+6%			−3.3%			+0.7%	

[a]Repeat measurements in males greater than 50 years of age who were studied at 0 and 12 months and who did not receive GH.

occurred in subjects 1, 4, and 5. These changes were not observed in the other two (2 and 3) or in the three controls. Change in bone density by dual photon absorptiometry techniques was not observed in any of the subjects.

Skin biopsy studies performed before treatment and after 6–12 months of GH treatment showed no change in collagen fibril diameter by electron microscopy in upper, mid-, and deep dermis; no change in collagen hydroxyproline or other amino acids to reflect changes in amount of collagen relative to other proteins; and that collagen types I, III, and V had no alteration in ratios after limited proteolysis with pepsin.

IV. DISCUSSION

The Sm-C determinations and GH secretion data from this study can be compared with data we recently published regarding these parameters in 10 young adult females, 10 young adult males, 8 postmenopausal adult females, and 8 males over 55 years of age (11). In the latter study there was a direct correlation of Sm-C concentrations with free estrogen concentrations in both sexes and an inverse relationship with the amount of GH secreted in pulses. Since we did not do estrogen determinations or GH pulsatility studies on the men and women in the study reported here, we can only speculate on why Sm-C concentrations did not change with age in females. Regardless, Sm-C determinations do decrease with age in males. Rudman et al. also reported that Sm-C determinations decrease in males with age (12). They reported values of 0.73 U/ml ± 0.04 for males 23–45 years of age and 0.41 U/ml ± 0.03 for those 52–87 years of age.

The secretion of GH occurred in fewer pulses with less amplitude in older males than in young males. We recently reported that there are fewer large pulses of GH in individuals of both sexes over the age of 50 (11). Specifically, both men and women over the age of 50 have decreased numbers of large high-amplitude pulses than young women, and significantly less of their GH is secreted in a pulsatile manner.

Older males are able to respond to short-term injections of GH with nitrogen retention, elevation of Sm-C, and increased calcium excretion. We reported similar studies previously (13), and we believe that GH therapy over a long period can enhance nitrogen and calcium balance in the elderly.

In keeping with the rises in Sm-C concentrations with the short-term injection of GH, the Sm-C determinations in the five males receiving GH over an extended period were maintained between 0.5 and 1.0 U for as long as 2 years (Figure 2). The dose of GH required to do this was 3.3 IU every other day. At this dose, the evidence for retention of significant amounts of total body nitrogen, potassium, and phosphorus and for calcium change is only suggestive.

Growth hormone at 3.3 IU every other day for 6–12 months did not change the characteristics of skin according to electron microscopy and biochemical analysis. The failure to observe changes might be related to dosage, but this seems unlikely because the Sm-C values were in the range of normal young adults. Possibly skin changes that occur with aging are irreversible.

V. CONCLUSION

From these and other studies we conclude that there are changes in the characteristics of GH production as aging occurs. However, details of the mechanisms for decreased GH are obscure. It is not clear whether GH injections will alter body composition, because it did not significantly affect the body composition of the limited number of males who received GH in this study. Additional studies using more subjects who receive larger doses of GH and/or GH over a longer period of time are needed.

ACKNOWLEDGMENTS

We gratefully acknowledge the collaboration of Ms. Sandra Jackson, Nursing Supervisor of the Clinical Research Center at the University of Virginia, and her staff; the assistance of Fotini Beziriannidis, Research Assistant; and the aid of Pamela Breeden, Executive Secretary, Department of Pediatrics, University of Virginia.

REFERENCES

1. Furlanetto RW, Underwood LE, Van Wyk JJ, D'Ercole AJ. Estimation of somatomedin-C levels in normals and patients with pituitary disease by radioimmunoassay. J. Clin. Invest. 60:648, 1977.

2. Copeland KC, Underwood LE, Van Wyk JJ. Induction of immunoreactive somatomedin-C in human serum by growth hormone. J. Clin. Endocrinol. Metab. 50:690, 1980.

3. Colbert C, Bachtell R. Radiographic absorptiometry. In Non-invasive Measurements of Bone Mass and Their Clinical Application, Cohn SH, ed., CRC Press, Boca Raton, FL, 1981.

4. Cohn S, Dombrowsky C. Absolute measurement of whole body potassium by gamma spectroscopy. J. Nucl. Med. 11:239, 1970.

5. Vaswani AN, Vartsky D, Ellis K, Yasmura S, Cohn S. Effects of caloric restriction on body composition and total body nitrogen as measured by neutron activation analysis. Int. Symp. Nucl. Activation Techniques Life Sci., Vienna, 1978. I AEA (Publ.) Sm-227/39, pp. 787–789.

6. Vaughn B, Boling E. Rapid assay procedures for tritium labelled water in body fluids. J. Lab. Clin. Med. 57:159, 1961.

7. Peppler W, Mazess R. Total body bone mineral and lean body mass by dual-photon absorptiometry. I. Theory and measurement procedure. Calc. Tissue Int. 33:353, 1981.

8. Sykes B, Luddle B, Frances M, Smith R. The estimation of two collagens from human dermis by interrupted electrophoresis. Biochem. Biophys. Res. Commun. 72:1472, 1976.

9. Light N, Bailey A. Covalent cross-links in collagen. Meth. Enzymol. 82(A):360–372, 1982.

10. Blizzard RM, Balian G, Nelson D, Savory J, Vaswani A, Aloia J, Cohn S, Johanson A, Sutphen E. The role of growth hormone (GH) in the aging process: The effect of GH administration on skin composition. (submitted)

11. Ho KY, Evans WS, Blizzard RM, Veldhuis JD, Merriam GR, Samojlik E, Furlanetto R, Rogol AD, Kaiser DL, Thorner MO. Effects of sex and

age on the 24 hour profile of GH secretion in man: An importance of endogenous estradiol concentrations. J. Clin. Invest. (in press)

12. Rudman D, Nagraj HS, Mattson DE, Ewe PR, Rudman IW. Hyposomatomedinemia in the nursing home patient. J. Am. Geriat. Soc. 34:427–430, 1986.

13. Bazzarre TL, Johanson AJ, Huseman CA, Varma MM, Blizzard RM. Human growth hormone changes with age. Proceedings of the Third International Symposium on Growth Hormone and Related Peptides, Milan, Excerpta Medica, Amsterdam, 1975.

12

Growth Hormone and Immunity

ARTHUR J. AMMANN

Genentech, Inc.
South San Francisco, California

There is abundant evidence to suggest bidirectional communication between the immune system and the (neuro)hormonal systems. Information has been derived from divergent studies including anatomic studies of the innervation of the thymus, lymph nodes and spleen; production of electrolytic lesions of the hypothalamus and assessment of the effects on organs of immunity; studies of the effects of hormones, neurotransmitters, and endorphins on the immune system; and evaluation of the effects of cytokines derived from immunologically competent cells on functions of the central nervous system.

I. INNERVATION OF LYMPHOID TISSUE

A number of studies suggest that stress and psychosocial events influence the response of the immune system and alter immunocompetence

(1–3). It is therefore of interest that direct innervation of lymphoid tissue, including thymus, lymph node, spleen, and bone marrow, has been demonstrated (4–6). Immunoreactive profiles in the thymus reveal the presence of vasoactive intestinal peptide, while the spleen shows Met-enkephalin-like, cholecystokinin-8-like, neurotensin-like, and neuropeptide Y-like immunoreactivity (4). Embryologically, the neural crest contributes to the development of the thymus and ablation of small portions of the neural crest result in abnormal thymus development (7). The presence of noradrenergic and peptidergic innervation of lymphoid tissue and the embryological contribution of the neural crest to thymus development suggests that there is a direct relationship between the immune system and the nervous system.

II. EFFECTS OF NEUROTRANSMITTERS AND NEUROHORMONES ON IMMUNE FUNCTION

Enkephalins and endorphins modulate immunological function in vitro and in vivo. β-Endorphin, Met-enkephalin, Leu-enkephalin, and morphine increase natural killer (NK) activity in vitro, an effect which can be inhibited with naloxone (8,9). Natural killer cells are cells that do not require prior sensitization to kill target cells, such as tumor cells. This effect may also occur in vivo as other investigators have shown that morphine, opioid forms of stress, and enkephalin administration decrease NK activity in vivo and increase susceptibility to malignancy (10,11).

T-cell mitogenic responses are enhanced in vivo by β-endorphin and enkephalins but are not affected by α-endorphin (12). In contrast, α-endorphin and enkephalins suppress antibody responses in vitro while β-endorphin has no effect (13).

Catecholamines may have a direct or indirect effect on immunological function. Adrenergic receptors (primarily β-adrenergic) are present on lymphocytes and may play a role in lymphocyte maturation and activity, perhaps by modulating cyclic AMP (14). A dual response to catecholamines is observed in vitro with stimulation of cytotoxic T-cells at low concentrations and inhibition at high concentrations (4).

Indirectly, catecholamines could alter traffic of lymphoid cells to and from organs by changing blood flow and thus modify the immune response.

Neuropeptides regulate the release of histamine and leukotrienes from mast cells. Neurotensin, substance P, somatostatin, as well as β-endorphin result in enhanced release of both histamine and leukotrienes in vitro and degranulation of mast cells in vivo (15). Substance P also stimulates T-lymphocyte mitogenesis as measured by ^{3}H-thymidine and ^{3}H-leucine uptake and enhances polymorphonuclear cell phagocytosis of yeast particles (16). Both somatostatin and vasoactive intestinal peptide cause a decrease of ^{3}H-thymidine and ^{3}H-leucine uptake by T-cells in vitro (6). Human lymphocytes have 23,000 to 35,000 receptors per cell for substance P or somatostatin and only 1700 for vasoactive intestinal peptide (16). The latter substance can activate adenylate cyclase in Molt lymphoblastic cell lines leading to cAMP-dependent protein kinase mediated phosphorylation of a Met-4b specific protein (17).

Two neurohypophyseal hormones, arginine vasopressin and oxytocin, are able to replace the requirement for T-cell growth factor (interleukin-2, IL-2) for T-cell mitogen-induced interferon-γ production (18). The arginine vasopressin activity was blocked by a competitive inhibitor while IL-2 activity remained intact, suggesting that arginine vasopressin acts on a receptor which is distinct from the IL-2 receptor.

III. NEUROANATOMIC LESIONS AND IMMUNE FUNCTION

The effects of bilateral electrolytic lesions in the anterior hypothalamus, hippocampus, or amygdala were studied in relation to effects on immune function. Control animals had lesions placed in the frontal lobes. Electrolytic lesions in the anterior hypothalamus resulted in decreased T-cell numbers, splenic mitogen responsiveness, antigen responsiveness, natural killer cell activity, and macrophage suppressor cell activity (19). Lesions in the hippocampus or amygdala decreased macrophage suppressor cell activity and increased splenic mitogen responsiveness. The mechanism whereby these effects are mediated is not understood.

IV. INTERACTIONS BETWEEN HORMONES AND THE IMMUNE SYSTEM

Cells of the immune system are known to produce and/or have receptors for several (neuro)hormones. Stimulated lymphocytes (virus infected) produce immunoreactive corticotropin (ACTH), which is biologically active in vitro and in vivo (20). Lymphocytes have high-affinity surface membrane receptors for ACTH which are associated with suppression of antibody responsiveness. Lymphocytes have also been shown to synthesize thytropin when stimulated by a T-cell mitogen (21).

Following activation of lymphocytes with the T-cell mitogen concanavalin A (Con-A), lymphocytes develop high-affinity surface membrane receptors for insulin (22). Similar receptors were demonstrated on T-cells activated by other mitogens or antigens and on B-cells activated by lipopolysaccharide (23,24). Thymocytes and the IM-9 human lymphocyte cell line have detectable and saturable cell surface receptors for GH (25,26). Additional studies indicate that both insulin and GH function as minor growth factors that potentiate lymphocyte activation (27).

A variety of immune cells have receptors for neurohormones on their membrane surface. Lymphoid cells possess receptors for enkephalins, neurotensin, somatostatin, substance P, and vasoactive intestinal peptide as well as opioids (17). Mast cells and polymorphonuclear cells have receptors for neurotensin and opioids (11,17).

Recently, immunoreactive oxytocin and neurophysin were identified in human thymus extracts. The amount of these neurohormones was in excess of the amount predicted from known concentrations of circulating hormone (28). Additionally, activation of murine T-helper cells was associated with the induction of abundant preproenkephalin mRNA synthesis (29).

Several additional hormones are known to regulate the immune response. Glucocorticoids inhibit the expression of macrophage Ia antigen and the production of IL-1 (30). Progesterone and estrogen are capable of inhibiting the rejection of grafts and are felt to be important immunoregulators during pregnancy (31). Orchidectomy increases thymus size, delays age-dependent involution of the thymus, and accelerates the spontaneous systemic lupus erythematosus observed in New

Zealand Black/New Zealand White (NB/NZW) male mice (32–34). In contrast, testosterone improves systemic lupus erythematosus in female NZB/ NZW mice while estrogen accelerates the disease in males (33,34).

V. EXPERIMENTAL EVIDENCE FOR A RELATIONSHIP BETWEEN GROWTH HORMONE AND THE IMMUNE SYSTEM

A relationship between GH and the immune system was first suggested in 1967 by two groups of investigators, one of which studied the effects of antibody to pituitary extracts on the thymus and lymphoid tissue, while the other studied the thymus and lymphoid tissue in the hereditary recessive pituitary dwarf mouse (Snell-Bagg) (35,36). Both investigators concluded that GH controls the growth of lymphoid tissue. Subsequently, delayed recovery of the total leukocyte count, antibody formation, and skin graft rejection was demonstrated in hypophysectomized adult rats (37). Additional effects of hypophysectomy include diminished NK cell function and decreased mean and maximum longevities in middle-aged mice (38,39).

Immunologic function was restored in the pituitary dwarf mouse by a combination of bovine somatotropic hormone and thyroxin consistent with the observation that both hormones are deficient in this animal model (40). Although more detailed studies of the endocrine system revealed that these mice were also deficient in leuteotropic hormone and ACTH, somatotropic hormone and thyroxine together were sufficient to restore immunologic function (40,41).

In a sex-linked dwarf chicken strain, bovine GH treatment resulted in enhanced antibody responses and bursal growth while thyroxine treatment stimulated thymus growth (42). Interestingly, neither treatment altered immune function in the autosomal dwarf chicken. Bovine growth hormone therapy alone partially restored immunologic function in immunodeficient Weimaraner dogs (43).

The relative ability of GH versus prolactin to restore deficient antibody responses in hypophysectomized rats was evaluated in several studies (44,45). Rat GH and rat prolactin were equally effective in restoring immunologic function.

VI. EVIDENCE FOR A RELATIONSHIP BETWEEN GROWTH HORMONE AND THE IMMUNE SYSTEM IN HUMANS

Evidence for clinically significant immunodeficiency disease in children with isolated GH deficiency has not been published. Nevertheless, several clinical studies indicate a relationship between GH deficiency and immunologic abnormalities, as well as a relationship between immunodeficiency disorders and other hormonal deficiencies.

Clinically significant immunodeficiency and hormone deficiency is found in patients with the DiGeorge syndrome, a disorder characterized by congenital heart disease, hypoparathyroidism, facial abnormalities, and immunodeficiency. The syndrome is the result of defective embryogenesis (46). Chronic mucocutaneous candidiasis may be associated with idiopathic endocrinology (Addison's disease, hypoparathyroidism, pernicious anemia) including ACTH deficiency (47). The disorder is felt to be a result of autoimmunity. In ataxia-telangiectasia, a syndrome associated with abnormal DNA repair, ovarian dysgenesis, testicular atrophy, and insulin resistance have been described (48).

In isolated GH deficiency, the response of peripheral blood lymphocytes to mitogen were normal (49,50). Increased B-cells, T-8 cells (suppressor), and decreased response to allogenic cells were described in a single study (50). In other studies, IL-2 production following mitogen stimulation was deficient and was not corrected following short-term GH therapy (51), while NK cell activity was reduced and could be corrected in vitro by GH (52). Deficiency of NK cell activity is the most consistent abnormality observed in GH deficiency and neuroendocrine abnormalities and has been described in hypophysectomized animals, animals with anatomic lesions of the hypothalamus, various forms of stress, and GH-deficient children (10,19,38,52–54).

VII. SUMMARY

Many studies provide evidence for a bidirectional communication between the immune system and (neuro)hormonal systems. Direct innervation of lymphoid tissue suggests a link between stimulation of the immune system and modulation of immunologic function. Neurotransmitters and neurohormones alter cytotoxic cell function, natural killer cell activity, and antibody formation. Neuropeptides regulate the release of pharmacologic agents from mast cells and neutrophils and can replace the cellular requirement for interleukin-2. Lymphocytes have receptors for ACTH and insulin on cell surface membranes and both glucocorticoids and sex hormones regulate immune responsiveness. Growth hormone deficiency has long been associated with immune abnormalities in animals but the relationship between growth hormone deficiency and decrease immunity in humans is less clear. However, in the aggregate, experimental evidence indicates there is a relationship between decreased growth hormone and altered immunity suggesting that continued investigations are necessary in both growth hormone–deficient children and aging adults.

REFERENCES

1. Plaut SM, Friedman SB. Psychosocial factors in infectious disease. In Psychoneuroimmunology, Ader R, ed., Academic Press, New York, 1981, pp. 3–14.

2. Sklar LS, Anisman H. Stress and coping factors influence tumor growth. Science 205:513–517, 1979.

3. Riley V. Psychoneuroendocrine influences on immunocompetence and neoplasia. Science 212:1100–1104, 1981.

4. Felten DL, Felten SY, Carlson SL, Olschowka JA, Livnat S. Noradrenergic and peptidergic innervation of lymphoid tissue. J. Immunol. 135:755–765, 1985.

5. Giron LT, Crutcher KA, Davis JN. Lymph nodes—A possible site for sympathetic neuronal regulation of immune responses. Ann. Neurol. 8:520–525, 1980.

6. Bulloch K, Pomerantz W. Autonomic nervous system innervation of thymic-related lymphoid tissue in wild-type and nude mice. J. Comp. Neurol. 228:57–68, 1984.

7. Bockman DE, Kirby ML. Neural crest interactions in the development of the immune system. J. Immunol. 135:766–768, 1985.

8. Mathews, PM, Froelich CJ, Sibbitt WL, Bankhurst AD. Enhancement of natural cytotoxicity by β-endorphin. J. Immunol. 130:1658–1662, 1983.

9. Wybran J. Enkephalins and endorphins as modifiers of the immune system: Present and future. Fed. Proc. 44:92–94, 1985.

10. Plotnikoff NP, Miller GC. Enkephalins as immunomodulators. Int. J. Immunopharmacol. 5:437–441, 1983.

11. Shavit Y, Terman GW, Martin FC, Lewis JW, Liebeskine JC, Gale RP. Stress, opioid peptides, the immune system, and cancer. J. Immunol. 135:834–837, 1985.

12. Gilman SC, Schwartz JM, Milner RJ, Bloom FE, Feldman JD. β-Endorphin enhances lymphocyte proliferative responses. Proc. Natl. Acad. Sci. USA 79:4226–4230, 1982.

13. Johnson HM, Smith EM, Torres BA, Blalock JE. Regulation of the *in vitro* antibody response by neuroendocrine hormones. Proc. Natl. Acad. Sci. USA 79:4171–4174, 1982.

14. Strom TB, Lundin AP, Carpenter CB. The role of cyclic nucleotides in lymphocyte activation and function. Prog. Clin. Immunol. 3:115–153, 1977.

15. Goetzl EJ, Chernov T, Frederic R, Payan DG. Neuropeptide regulation of the expression of immediate hypersensitivity. J. Immunol. 135:802–805, 1985.

16. Payan DG, Goetzl EJ. Modulation of lymphocyte function by sensory neuropeptides. J. Immunol. 135:783–786, 1985.

17. O'Dorisio MS, Wood CL, O'Dorisio TM. Vasoactive intestinal peptide and neuropeptide modulation of the immune response. J. Immunol. 135:792–796, 1985.

18. Johnson HM, Torres BA. Regulation of lymphokine production by arginine vasopressin and oxytocin: Modulation of lymphocyte function by neurohypophyseal hormones. J. Immunol. 135:773–775, 1985.

19. Roszman TL, Jackson JC, Cross RJ, Titus MJ, Markesbery WR, Brooks WH. Neuroanatomic and neurotransmitter influences on immune function. J. Immunol. 135:769–772, 1985.

20. Smith EM, Harbour-McMenamin D, Blalock JE. Lymphocyte produc-

tion of endorphins and endorphin-mediated immunoregulatory activity. J. Immunol. 135:779–782, 1985.

21. Smith EM, Phan M, Kruger TE, Coppenhaver DH, Blalock JE. Human lymphocyte production of immunoreactive thyrotropin. Proc. Natl. Acad. Sci. USA 80:6010–6013, 1983.

22. Krug U, Krug F, Cuatrecasas P. Emergence of insulin receptors on human lymphocytes during *in vitro* transformation. Proc. Natl. Acad. Sci. USA 69:2604–2608, 1972.

23. Helderman JH, Reynolds TC, Strom TB. The insulin receptor as a universal marker of activated lymphocytes. Eur. J. Immunol. 8:589–595, 1978.

24. Helderman JH. T cell cooperation for the genesis of B cell insulin receptors. J. Immunol. 131:644–650, 1983.

25. Arrembrecht S. Specific binding of growth hormone to thymocytes. Nature 252:255–257, 1974.

26. Lesniak MA, Gordon P, Roth J, Gavin JR. Binding of ^{125}I-human growth hormone to specific receptors in human cultured lymphocytes. J. Biol. Chem. 249:1661–1667, 1974.

27. Snow EC. Insulin and growth hormone function as minor growth factors that potentiate lymphocyte activation. J. Immunol. 135:776–778, 1985.

28. Geenen V, Legros J-J, Franchimont P, Baudrihaye M, Defresne M-P, Boniver J. The neuroendocrine thymus: Coexistence of oxytocin and neurophysin in the human thymus. Science 232:508–511, 1986.

29. Zurawski G, Benedik M, Kamb BJ, Abrams JS, Zurawski SM, Lee FD. Activation of mouse T-helper cells induces abundant preproenkephalin mRNA synthesis. Science 232:772–775, 1986.

30. Dinarello CA. Interleukin-1. Rev. Infect. Dis. 6:51–95, 1984.

31. Wyle FA, Kent JR. Immunosuppression by sex steroid hormones. I. The effect upon PHA- and PPD-stimulated lymphocytes. Clin. Exp. Immunol. 27:407–415, 1977.

32. Dumont F, Barrois R, Habbersett RC. Prepubertal orchidectomy induces thymic abnormalities in aging (NZB × SJL)F_1 male mice. J. Immunol. 129:1642–1648, 1982.

33. Roubinian JR, Papoian R, Talal N. Androgenic hormones modulate autoantibody responses and improve survival in Murine lupus. J. Clin. Invest. 59:1066–1070, 1977.

34. Melez KA, Attallah AM, Harrison ET, Reveche ES. TI immune abnormalities in the diabetic New Zealand obese (NZO) mouse: Insulin treatment partially suppresses splenic hyperactivity measured by flow cytometric analysis. Clin. Immunol. Immunopathol. 36:110, 1985.

35. Pierpaoli W, Sorkin E. Nature 215:834, 1967.

36. Baroni C. Experientia 23:282, 1967.

37. Duquesnoy RJ, Mariani T, Good RA. Effect of hypophysectomy on immunological recovery after sublethal irradiation of adult rats. Proc. Soc. Exp. Biol. Med. 131:1176–1178, 1969.

38. Cross RJ, Markesbery WR, Brooks WH, Roszman TL. Hypothalamic-immune interactions: Neuromodulation of natural killer activity by lesioning of the anterior hypothalamus. Immunology 51:399–405, 1984.

39. Harrison DE, Archer JR, Astle CM. The effect of hypophysectomy on thymic aging in mice. J. Immunol. 129:2673–2677, 1982.

40. Baroni CD, Fabris N, Bertoli G. Effects of hormones on development and function of lymphoid tissues. Immunol. 17:303–314, 1969.

41. Fabris N, Pierpaoli W, Sorkin E. Hormones and the immunological capacity. Clin. Exp. Immunol. 9:227–240, 1971.

42. Marsh JA, Gause WC, Sandhu S, Scanes CG. Enhanced growth and immune development in dwarf chickens treated with mammalian growth hormone and thyroxine. Proc. Soc. Exp. Biol. Med. 175:351–360, 1984.

43. Roth JA, Kaeberle ML, Grier RL, Hopper JG, Spiegel HE. McAllister HA. Improvement in clinical condition and thymus morphologic features associated with growth hormone treatment of immunodeficient dwarf dogs. Ann. J. Vet. Res. 45:1151–1155, 1984.

44. Fabris N, Pierpaoli W, Sorkin E. Hormones and the immunological capacity. IV. Restorative effects of developmental hormones or of lymphocytes on the immunodeficiency syndrome of the dwarf mouse. Clin. Exp. Immunol. 9:227–240, 1971.

45. Nagy E, Berczi I, Friesen HG. Regulation of immunity in rats by lactogenic and growth hormones. Acta. Endocrinol. 102:351–357, 1983.

46. DiGeorge AM. Congenital absence of the thymus and its immunologic consequences: Concurrence with congenital hypoparathyroidism. In Immunologic Deficiency Diseases in Man, Bergsma D, Good RA, eds., National Foundation: Birth Defects Orig. Art Ser., Vol. 4, No. 1, Williams and Wilkins, Baltimore, 1968, pp. 116–123.

47. Castells S, Fikrig S, Inamdar S, Orti E. Familial moniliasis, defective delayed hypersensitivity, and adrenocorticotropic hormone deficiency. J. Pediat. 79:72–79, 1971.

48. Ammann AJ, DuQuesnoy RJ, Good RA. Endocrinological studies in ataxia-telangiectasia and other immunological deficiency diseases. Clin. Exp. Immunol. 6:587–595, 1969.

49. Abbassi V, Bellanti JA. Humoral and cell-mediated immunity in growth hormone-deficient children: Effect of therapy with human growth hormone. Pediat. Res. 19:299–301, 1985.

50. Gupta S, Fikrig SM, Noval MS. Immunological studies in patients with isolated growth hormone deficiency. Clin. Exp. Immunol. 54:87–90, 1983.

51. Rapaport R, Oleske J, Schenkman S, Churchill J, Kirkpatrick C. Growth hormone deficiency: Interleukin 2 and immune function. Pediat. Res. 19:612, 1985. (abstract)

52. Kiess W, Doerr H, Butenandt O, Belohradsky BH. Lymphocyte subsets and natural-killer activity in growth hormone deficiency. N. Engl. J. Med. 314:321, 1986.

53. Roder JC, Pross HF. The biology of the human natural killer cell. J. Clin. Immunol. 2:249–263, 1982.

54. Denckla WD. Interactions between age and the neuroendocrine and immune systems. Fed. Proc. 37:1263–1267, 1978.

13

Growth Hormone in the Surgical Patient

JAMES MANSON*
and DOUGLAS W. WILMORE†

Harvard Medical School
and Brigham and Women's Hospital
Boston, Massachusetts

I. THE METABOLIC RESPONSE TO STRESS

The classic studies of Cuthbertson performed in Glasgow in the 1930s and the more recent work of Moore in Boston established that the body's response to operation, injury, and infection involves not merely a local healing process, but also a systemic metabolic response. This response is orchestrated by the central nervous system and mediated by neural and

Current affiliations:
*University Hospital of South Manchester, Manchester, England.
†Brigham and Women's Hospital, Boston, Massachusetts.

hormonal factors, with additional regulation from substances released from circulating and fixed macrophages (e.g., lymphokines).

One feature of the metabolic adaptation observed following stress is the mobilization of amino acids from skeletal muscle, the major site of body protein. These compounds are transported to visceral organs, where they serve as precursors of acute phase proteins and new glucose. The nitrogen released from the amino acids forms urea, which is excreted in the urine. Nitrogen excretion is a consistent feature of the metabolic response to stress, and the amount lost generally is proportional to the severity of the insult (Table 1).

Increased net proteolysis occurs following most major surgical procedures. The protein losses are minimal and well tolerated if the patient is healthy, body composition is normal, and the clinical course uncomplicated. Following major burn injury, multiple trauma, or prolonged sepsis, however, continued erosion of body protein and progressive loss of body nitrogen occur and result in protein malnutrition. In this situation the patient is unable to heal wounds and/or resist infection. Ultimately, recovery may be jeopardized. Because there is no stored protein, loss of body nitrogen through uncontrolled protein catabolism will eventually result in a functional deficit.

Table 1. Estimates of Cumulative Nitrogen Loss Following Catabolic Illness (first 10 days, ad libitum feeding)

Precipitating factor	Cumulative nitrogen loss (g)
Major burn	170
Multiple injury	150
Peritonitis	136
Simple fracture	115
Major operation	50
Minor operation	24
Typhoid fever (untreated)	116
Pneumonia (untreated)	59

Source: Ref. 58.

II. THE ROLE OF NUTRITIONAL SUPPORT

Nutrient provision alters the catabolic response to stress. Administration of adequate protein and calories can decrease or even abolish the negative nitrogen balance seen in the posttraumatic state (1,2). Clinical trials have evaluated the effect of perioperative feeding in patients undergoing major surgery. Some suggest that nutrient administration reduces mortality and morbidity associated with operation (3,4), but others have not (5). Studies of protein turnover, synthesis, and catabolism demonstrate that feeding critically ill patients does not alter the accelerated rate of protein breakdown. Rather, food intake increases protein synthesis, which reduces the *net* loss of body protein (6). In addition, specialized nutritional support is associated with its own set of complications, which are generally related to the use of feeding tubes or central venous catheters. Further, patients may be paralyzed while receiving assisted ventilation or may have severe renal or hepatic impairment. In many instances even the most carefully planned and expertly administered nutritional regime may not result in nitrogen equilibrium or restoration of body protein.

III. MODIFYING THE METABOLIC RESPONSE TO STRESS

The deleterious effects of continued erosion of body protein following surgery or injury, especially when associated with sepsis, have led investigators to examine the possibility of modifying the metabolic response to stress. Various approaches have been utilized. Physicians have increased ambient temperature to minimize cold stress and administered prostaglandin inhibitors in an attempt to reduce the elevated thermoregulatory set point which occurs following stress. The hormonal balance in the posttraumatic phase favors catabolism, and elevated circulating levels of the "counterregulatory" hormones glucagon, cortisol, and the catecholamines have been observed consistently. Although serum insulin concentrations are normal or raised slightly, peripheral tissues (particularly muscle) exhibit insulin resistance and insulin's effects on glucose transport are blunted (7). Exogenous insulin has been administered in an attempt to decrease nitrogen losses after injury (8,9), and anabolic steroids have also been employed (10,11). Administration of these agents was associated with nitrogen retention but neither approach has become applicable because of potentially deleterious side effects.

IV. GROWTH HORMONE

Physiological Properties

Growth hormone (GH) stimulates protein synthesis, whether this is assessed by increased uptake of labeled amino acid into cells (12) or by the accretion of body protein measured by compositional analysis (13, 20). Many of the growth-promoting actions of GH are mediated by an intermediary polypeptide hormone, insulinlike growth factor I (IGF-I), also referred to as somatomedin C (Sm-C) (14). In addition, GH has a "pancreatotopic" effect and augments insulin production (15). GH also stimulates lipolysis, raises serum fatty acid concentrations (16), and increases fat oxidation (17,20). GH also promotes ketogenesis, which may be a direct effect of the hormone and not merely a result of increased fat metabolization (18,19). Animal experiments have demonstrated that chronic administration of GH spares protein and utilizes fat stores (20,21).

As a result of these properties GH has been considered a potent anabolic agent to offset posttraumatic protein catabolism. Now that biosynthetic GH is available in unlimited quantities, there is renewed interest in GH therapy in catabolic surgical patients.

The Effect of Growth Hormone on Stress

Growth hormone is released from the anterior pituitary gland in response to traumatic injury (22), burn trauma (23), surgical operation (24,25), infectious disease (26), and administration of endotoxin (27). Carey and colleagues examined serum GH levels following severe trauma in military personnel in Vietnam (22). The average serum concentration of GH in seriously injured soldiers arriving at the medical base was 58.8 ng/ml, and the level in two soldiers who did not respond to treatment and died soon afterward was more than 400 ng/ml.

Reports (24,25) have confirmed the prompt but relatively short-lived elevation in GH following a surgical procedure: concentrations return to normal approximately four to seven days following operation. Wright and Johnston (24) demonstrated that the rise in serum GH was proportional to the severity of the operation.

The role of GH in stress states was examined by Dahn et al., who determined the response of GH following administration of an intravenous glucose load in 13 seriously ill patients (28). They found that some patients responded by markedly increasing GH concentration (mean 400%), and others demonstrated only a moderate response (mean 140%). The patients who were otherwise comparable could be divided into two groups on the basis of their GH responses. The "hyper-responders" had significantly lower plasma concentrations of amino acids despite similar splanchnic amino acid exchange, suggesting that net proteolysis was decreased. In addition, the "responders" had a significantly higher helper-to-suppressor T-cell subpopulation ratio, supporting work by others indicating that GH may augment immune responses. Those patients with a moderate response following the intravenous glucose load were more catabolic and demonstrated greater immunosuppression than the GH responding group. The authors concluded that the ability to mount a GH response in stress states is beneficial and aids patient recovery.

Other investigations have demonstrated that GH production, as determined by integrating the response curve following a standard provocative stimulus, decreases with age (34,35). In addition, IGF-I concentrations decline with age but respond to injection of exogenous GH (36). Although no studies relate GH elaboration in stress states to age, it might be deduced that elderly patients, who make up the majority of individuals undergoing major elective surgery, might have blunted GH responses. This group of patients may particularly benefit from GH administration.

Investigations of the changes in serum IGF-I concentrations following musculoskeletal trauma (29,30) and burn injury (31) demonstrate that IGF-I levels fall immediately following injury and return to

normal after 1–2 weeks. This decrease in IGF-I occurs at the time GH
levels rise. The posttraumatic dissociation of the normal relationship
between GH and IGF-I also occurs in starvation (32) and in poorly
controlled diabetes (33), where IGF-I concentrations tend to be low
despite elevated serum levels of GH. The reason for this dissociation
of the usual relationship is not clear, but it may be a physiological
mechanism acting in an environment where protein conservation is not
a priority for the organism, but high levels of GH are useful to maintain circulating glucose levels and aid in the mobilization of fat.

Exogenous Growth Hormone Administration in
Catabolic States

In 1941 Cuthbertson et al. compared the responses of control rats to a
group of rats treated with crude anterior pituitary extract following
femoral fracture (37). The rats receiving pituitary extract excreted
significantly less urinary nitrogen than untreated controls, and weight
loss was almost completely abolished. Fifteen years later, Prudden and
co-workers gave bovine growth hormone (BGH) for 5 days to four burn
patients and compared nitrogen balance to a period in which no GH was
given in the same individuals (38). They observed that BGH improved
nitrogen balance only when a certain amount of nitrogen was ingested
(deemed the ''critical level''); when protein intake was inadequate the
hormone increased the catabolic response. In addition, BGH treatment
improved protein conservation only late in the postburn period during
convalescence, rather than early during the catabolic period. Pearson et
al. (39) analyzed the mineral balance data from the same patients and
reported similar responses in potassium balance.
  In 1961 Liljedahl and colleagues gave hGH to a group of severely
burned patients, relatively soon after the burn injury (40). The subjects
were allowed food intake ad libitum. Growth hormone improved nitrogen balance; this response was due both to increased food intake (nitrogen intake) and to decreased urinary nitrogen losses. Similar alterations were observed in the balance of phosphorus and potassium.
Albumin concentrations rose during GH treatment and albumin catabolism decreased.

These very encouraging results were partly confirmed in 1967 by Soroff et al., who administered hGH to burn patients receiving a constant diet (41). They reported that GH improved nitrogen and mineral retention in the later, "anabolic phase " of injury (after nitrogen balance had already become positive). This study also confirmed the lipolytic effects of GH; respiratory quotient (RQ) fell in six of the nine studies following GH treatment. These results were different from earlier studies by the same group using BGH, where no beneficial effect was observed (42).

The most recent work in burn patients was performed by Wilmore and co-workers in 1974 (43). With patients acting as their own controls, these investigators demonstrated a significant decrease in nitrogen losses following GH administration in 9 of the 10 patients studied. All individuals received adequate protein and caloric feedings. Growth hormone administration resulted in significant increase in basal insulin concentration and augmented insulin responses following an intravenous glucose load. They described a highly significant relationship among nitrogen intake, nitrogen balance, and basal insulin concentrations. These findings stressed the importance of the insulinotropic effect of GH in mediating nitrogen retention (Figure 1).

The action of GH following elective operations has not been studied extensively. Johnston and Hadden administered hGH to four patients undergoing herniorraphy but were unable to demonstrate any effect on nitrogen metabolism (44). Ward, Halliday, and Sim administered biosynthetic GH for six days to patients following major gastrointestinal surgery (45). These patients received 400 kcal/day as dextrose infusion; no exogenous amino acids were administered. Growth hormone caused significant nitrogen retention and increases in serum insulin and IGF-I concentrations. Growth hormone treatment was also associated with an increase in protein turnover. When protein synthesis was expressed as a percentage of breakdown the patients receiving GH demonstrated greater synthesis when compared to controls.

We have investigated the effect of hGH in normal volunteers receiving parenteral nutrition for periods of 6 days to study the effects of GH during hypocaloric feeding. Each period was separated by at least 2 weeks. During one period the subjects received 10 mg daily of

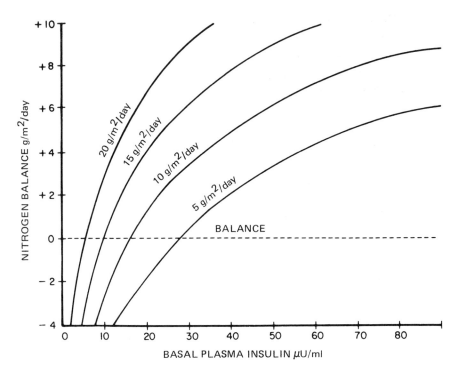

Figure 1. Nitrogen balance becomes more positive as insulin concentrations rise and as the quantity of nitrogen (i.e., protein) in the diet increases. On a fixed food intake, GH increases the plasma levels of insulin. $y = -19.97 + 5.21 \, \mathrm{Log_e} \, BI + 0.56 \, N_{IN}$. y = nitrogen balance (g/m²/day). BI = basal insulin (μU/ml). N_{IN} = nitrogen intake (g/m²/day). $r^2 = 0.76$; $p < 0.05$. (From Ref. 43.)

GH subcutaneously, and during the other period they received saline injections (46). Because we were particularly interested in the feedings, we administered one of three levels of energy to those subjects— adequate (basal metabolic energy requirements +25%), 50% of adequate energy requirements, and only 30% of adequate needs. Adequate dietary nitrogen was provided at a constant note during all studies.

Growth hormone administration produced positive nitrogen balance at all levels of energy intake (Figure 2). This occurred at the

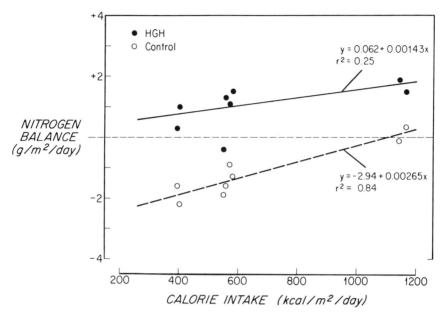

Figure 2. In normal individuals, nitrogen balance is negative during hypocaloric feedings and approaches equilibrium when adequate calories ($\cong 1100$–1200 kcal/m²/day) are administered. Nitrogen balance remained positive during GH administration, even when only 30–50% of energy requirements were provided.

lowest energy intake where the only nonprotein calorie source was approximately 140 grams of dextrose per day. Positive potassium and phosphorus balance occurred in association with the nitrogen retention. These three elements were retained in proportions corresponding to their relative amounts found in skeletal muscle, suggesting strongly that the nitrogen retained was in the form of muscle tissue.

Nitrogen retention was accompanied by increased serum insulin concentrations and augmented insulin production as assessed by C-peptide excretion. Increased ketone excretion and elevated serum levels of lipid substrates also occurred. Serum IGF-I increased following GH administration. On the final day of each study period the response to a 100-g oral glucose load was assessed by simultaneous measurement of respiratory gas exchange and substrate forearm flux over a 4-hour period. Despite a greatly increased insulin response to the glucose load, GH produced significantly lower forearm (and derived whole body) muscle glucose uptake. However, glucose oxidation calculated from gas exchange measurements did not change with GH treatment, suggesting that other tissues adequately metabolized the glucose administered.

These results suggest that in normal individuals, the anabolic effects of GH are not dependent on an adequate energy intake.

V. SPECIFIC CONSIDERATIONS FOR GROWTH HORMONE THERAPY IN CATABOLIC SURGICAL PATIENTS

Ability to Induce Insulinlike Growth Factor I Production

Froesch et al. (47) emphasized the difference between the production, storage, and release of insulin and IGF-I. Insulin is synthesized in the islets of Langerhans and stored in granules, which are released into the blood by exocytosis in response to a rise in blood glucose. IGF-I occurs in larger quantities in the serum than in any other tissue. It apparently does not occur in a stored form but is synthesized by the hepatocytes in response to GH stimulation (48). As previously discussed, a close correlation exists between GH and IGF-I levels in normals. This relationship does not occur during malnutrition, uncontrolled diabetes, and following injury (30,32,33). Thus provision of GH may not induce IGF-I production in all clinical situations. IGF-I is produced largely in the liver (48), and its elaboration is also reduced in liver disease (49). Severely ill patients, particularly those with liver dysfunction, may not be able to mount an IGF-I response to GH therapy, although this remains to be examined in a controlled study. Presumably the anabolic consequences of the insulinotropic and the lipolytic/ketogenic properties of GH would persist if IGF-I levels were not elevated, but promotion of protein synthesis would be limited.

Hyperglycemia

Despite its insulinotropic effect, GH administration is associated with glucose intolerance secondary to decreased uptake of glucose into peripheral tissue (50,51). Growth hormone also may act to oppose the central effect of insulin by decreasing hepatic gluconeogenesis. Experimental evidence on this point is contradictory (51–53).

In the studies on catabolic patients described earlier and on work on normal volunteers, hyperglycemia was not observed. However, there remains a concern that certain patients who exhibit insulin resistance related to their disease process will become markedly glucose intolerant following GH administration. This hyperglycemia would be accentuated if hypertonic glucose solutions were administered by the intravenous route.

Dosage, Route of Administration, and Timing

In their study in burn patients, Wilmore et al. (43) gave a fixed GH dose of 10 mg/day. When this was converted to milligrams per kilogram of body weight for each patient, a significant positive correlation was observed between dose and quantity of nitrogen retained. Dose–response relationships, however, have not been evident in studies of GH treatment in the posttraumatic state, possibly because GH has to be given over the narrow range between 5 and 10 mg (10 and 20 IU) per day. In our study on normal volunteers, marked changes in nitrogen and mineral balances were achieved with 10 mg (20 IU) per day. It is not known what effects would occur with lower doses and these data are needed.

Traditionally, GH has been administered by intramuscular injections to hypopituitary dwarfs. The subcutaneous route has been avoided because it was believed it might predispose to the formation of antibodies. Recent studies (54,55) have been unable to confirm this suspicion. Both routes of administration are equivalent in terms of peak and integrated serum concentrations of GH, IGF-I response, and linear growth rate. The subcutaneous route, which was used in our normal volunteers, is less painful. However, intravenous GH administration is the ideal route of administration, particularly in patients receiving intravenous feedings. The efficacy of this route of administration awaits detailed study.

In the work of Wilmore et al. (43) and Ward et al. (45), GH was given in the early evening so that the increase in serum concentrations would mirror the physiological rise in GH that occurs during sleep. In our work on normal volunteers and in most other studies on burn patients, GH was injected in the morning. A controlled comparison of these two types of administration has not been conducted. Available evidence suggests that the effect of exogenously administered GH would be greater at a later rather than earlier stage in recovery following injury or operation, when endogenous production of GH is low.

VI. POTENTIAL APPLICATIONS OF GROWTH HORMONE THERAPY IN SURGICAL PATIENTS

If our findings in normal volunteers can be extended to catabolic patients and the results of Ward et al. (45) in the postoperative state are confirmed by other workers, peripheral venous feedings containing adequate nitrogen but inadequate calories administered with GH may offer an alternative method of therapy to central venous feedings in patients with adequate fat stores. Thus nitrogen balance could be achieved without relying on the complexities of central vein hypercaloric nutrition.

In patients with poor cardiopulmonary reserve or renal failure it is sometimes difficult to provide adequate nutrition because of the need to restrict fluids. Growth hormone therapy could optimize the impact of the protein administered and might exert other beneficial effects. In hypercatabolic patients receiving large quantities of calories and protein, GH therapy might decrease nitrogen losses and aid in the attainment of positive nitrogen balance.

However, the most appealing aspect of this approach is the lipolytic response to GH therapy. The metabolic response allows patients to utilize their own fat stores, but at the same time synthesize protein. This shift in fuel utilization together with reports of appetite stimulation may facilitate rebuilding of lean body mass at a time usually associated with protein wasting. It is unknown if such a process would shorten convalescence and aid recovery following catabolic illness, but this thesis should be tested.

It also has been demonstrated in animal experiments that GH is a potent stimulator of wound healing, as measured by wound strength and rate of wound closure (56,57). Growth hormone may have a role in stimulating wound healing in selected patients, and the possibility exists that this action may extend to the acceleration of fistula closure, burn wound healing, and bone repair. Such effects would have profound implications on patient care. Controlled trials of GH therapy need to be performed to determine effects of GH on patient outcome and to identify those patients who might profit from this therapy. The availability of GH and other growth factors, as a result of rDNA technology, holds great promise for improved care of catabolic surgical patients.

REFERENCES

1. Moghissi K, Hornshaw J, Teasdale PR, Dawes EA. Parenteral nutrition in carcinoma of the esophagus treated by surgery: Nitrogen balance and clinical studies. Br. J. Surg. 64:125–128, 1977.

2. Wesley-Alexander J, Macmillan BG, Stinnett JD, et al. Beneficial effects of aggressive protein feeding in severely burned children. Ann. Surg. 192: 505–517, 1980.

3. Muller JM, Brenner U, Dienst C, Pichlmaier H. Preoperative parenteral feeding in patients with gastrointestinal carcinoma. Lancet 1:68–71, 1982.

4. Young GA, Hill LH. A controlled study of protein-sparing therapy after excision of the rectum. Ann. Surg. 192:183–191, 1980.

5. Holter AR, Rosen HM, Fischer JE. The effects of hyperalimentation on major surgery in patients with malignant disease: A prospective study. Arch. Chir. Scand. 466(Supp.):86–87, 1977.

6. Herrman VM, Clark D, Wilmore DW, Moore ED. Protein metabolism: Effect of disease and altered intake on the stable N curve. Surg. Forum 31:92–94, 1980.

7. Brooks DC, Bessey PQ, Black PR, Aoki TT, Wilmore DW. Post-traumatic insulin resistance in uninjured forearm tissue. J. Surg. Res. 37:100–107, 1984.

8. Hinton P, Allison SP, Littlejohn S, Lloyd J. Insulin and glucose to reduce catabolic response to injury in burned patients. Lancet i:767–769, 1971.

9. Woolfson AMJ, Heatley RV, Allison SP. Insulin to inhibit protein catabolism after injury. N. Engl. J. Med. 300:14–17, 1979.

10. Tweedle D, Walton C, Johnston IDA. The effect of an anabolic steroid on postoperative nitrogen balance. Br. J. Clin. Prac. 27:130–132, 1973.

11. Michelsen CB, Askanasi J, Kinney JM, Gump FE, Elwyn DH. Effect of an anabolic steroid on nitrogen balance and amino acid patterns after total hip replacement. J. Trauma, 22:410–413, 1982.

12. Kostyo JL. In vitro effects of growth hormone and corticotropin on amino acid transport in muscle. Acta Endocrinol. 51(supp.):943, 1960.

13. Collipp PJ, Curti V, Thomas J, et al. Body composition changes in children receiving human growth hormone. Metabolism 22:589, 1973.

14. Salmon WD Jr, Daughaday WH. A hormonally controlled serum factor which stimulates sulfate incorporation by cartilage in vitro. J. Lab. Clin. Med. 49:825–835, 1957.

15. Anselmino KJ, Herold L, Hoffman FR. Uber die pankreatrope witkung von hypophysendvorderlappenextrakten. Klin. Wrsch. 12(2):1245–1247, 1933.

16. Raben MS, Hollenberg CH. Effect of growth hormone on plasma free fatty acids. J. Clin. Invest. 38:484–488, 1959.

17. Gaebler OH. Some effects of anterior pituitary extracts on nitrogen metabolism, waste balance and energy metabolism. J. Exp. Med. 57:349–363, 1933.

18. Greenbaum AL, McLean P. The influence of pituitary growth hormone on the catabolism of fat. Biochem. J. 54:413–424, 1953.

19. Shipley RA, Long CNH. Studies on the ketogenic activity of the anterior pituitary. J. Biochem. 22:2242–2256, 1938.

20. Korenchevsky V. The influence of the hypophysis on metabolism,

growth and sexual organs of male rats and rabbits. Biochem. J. 24:383–393, 1930.

21. Greenbaum AL. Changes in body composition and respiratory quotient of adult female rats treated with purified growth hormone. Biochem. J. 54:400–407, 1953.

22. Carey LC, Cloutier CT, Lowery BD. Growth hormone and adrenocortical response to shock and trauma in the human. Ann. Surg. 174:451–460, 1971.

23. Wilmore DW, Orcutt TW, Mason AD, Pruitt BA Jr. Alterations in hypothalamic function following thermal injury. J. Trauma 15:697–703, 1975.

24. Wright PD, Johnston IDA. The effect of surgical operation on growth hormone levels in plasma. Surgery 77:479–486, 1975.

25. Aarima M, Syvalahti E, Viikari J, Ovaska J. Insulin, growth hormone and catecholamines as regulators of energy metabolism in the course of surgery. Acta Chir. Scand. 144:411–422, 1978.

26. Beisel WR, Woeber KA, Bartelloni PJ, Ingbar SH. Growth hormone response during sandfly fever. J. Clin. Endocrinol. Metab. 28:1220–1221, 1968.

27. Frohman LA, Horton ES, Lebovitz HE. Growth hormone releasing action of a pseudomonas endotoxin. Metabolism 16:57–67, 1967.

28. Dahn MS, Mitchell RA, Smith S, et al. Altered immunologic function and nitrogen metabolism associated with depression of plasma growth hormone. JPEN 8:690–694, 1984.

29. Coates CL, Burwell RG, Carlin SA, et al. The somatomedin activity in plasma from patients with multiple mechanical injuries with observations on plasma cortisol. Injury 13:100–107, 1981.

30. Frayn KN, Price DA, Maycock PF, Carroll SM. Plasma somatomedin activity after injury in man and its relationship to other hormonal and metabolic changes. Clin. Endocrinol. 20:179–187, 1984.

31. Coates CL, Burwell RG, Carlin SA, et al. Somatomedin activity in plasma from burned patients with observations on plasma cortisol. Burns 7:425–433, 1981.

32. Grant DB, Hambley J, Becker D, et al. Reduced sulfation factor in undernourished children. Arch. Dis. Child. 48:596–600, 1973.

33. Winter RJ, Phillips LS, Klein MN, et al. Somatomedin activity and diabetic control in children with insulin-dependent diabetes. Diabetes 28:952–954, 1979.

34. Bazzare TL, et al. Human growth hormone changes with age. Proceedings of the Third International Symposium on Growth Hormone and Related Peptides, Milan, September 1975, Excerpta Medica, Amsterdam, 1976.

35. Finkelstein JW, Roffwarg HP, Boyar RM, et al. Age-related change in the 24-hour spontaneous secretion of growth hormone. J. Clin. Endocrinol. Metab. 35:665, 1972.

36. Johanson AJ, Blizzard RM. Low somatomedin-C levels in older men rise in response to growth hormone administration. Johns Hopkins Med. J. 149:115–117, 1981.

37. Cuthbertson DP, Shaw GB, Young FG. The influence of anterior pituitary extract on the metabolic response of the rat to injury. J. Endocrinol. 2:468–474, 1941.

38. Prudden JF, Pearson E, Soroff HS. Studies on growth hormone. II: The effect on the nitrogen metabolism of severely burned patients. Surg. Gyn. Obs. 102:695–701, 1956.

39. Pearson E, Soroff HS, Prudden JF, Schwarz MS. Studies on growth hormone. V: Effect on the mineral and nitrogen balances of burned patients. Am. J. Med. Sci. 239:17–25, 1960.

40. Liljedahl S-O, Gemzell C-A, Plantin L-O, Birke G. Effect of human growth hormone in patients with severe burns. Acta Chir. Scand. 122: 1–14, 1961.

41. Soroff HS, Rozin RR, Mooty JM, et al. Role of human growth hormone in the response to trauma: I. Metabolic effects following burns. Ann. Surg. 166:739–752, 1967.

42. Soroff HS, Pearson E, Green NL, Artz CP. The effect of growth hormone on nitrogen balance at various levels of intake in burned patients. Surg. Gyn. Obs. 111:259–273, 1960.

43. Wilmore DW, Moylan JA, Bristow BF, Mason AD, Pruitt BA Jr.

Anabolic effects of human growth hormone and high caloric feedings following thermal injury. Surg. Gyn. Obs. 138:875–884, 1974.

44. Johnston IDA, Hadden DR. Effect of human growth hormone on the metabolic response to surgical trauma. Lancet 1:584–586, 1963.

45. Ward HC, Halliday D, Sim AW. Protein and energy metabolism with biosynthetic human growth hormone after gastrointestinal surgery. Data presented at ESPEN meeting, Milan, 1984. (unpublished)

46. Manson J McK, Wilmore DW. Positive nitrogen balance with human growth hormone and hypocaloric intravenous feeding. Surgery 100:188–197, 1986.

47. Froesch ER, Schmid C, Schwander J, Zapf J. Actions of insulin-like growth factors. Ann. Rev. Physiol. 47:443–467, 1985.

48. Schwander J, Hauri C, Zapf J, Froesch ER. Synthesis and secretion of insulin-like growth factor and its binding protein by the perfused rat liver: Dependence on growth hormone status. Endocrinology 113:297–305, 1983.

49. Wu A, Grant DB, Hambley J, Levi AJ. Reduced serum somatomedin activity in patients with chronic liver disease. Clin. Sci. Mol. Med. 47:359–366, 1974.

50. Rizza RA, Mandarino LJ, Gerich JE. Effects of growth hormone on insulin action in man. Diabetes 31:663–669, 1982.

51. Cheng JS, Kalant N. Effects of insulin and growth hormone on the flux rates of plasma glucose and plasma free fatty acids in man. J. Clin. Endocrinol. 31:647–653, 1970.

52. Bratusch-Marrain PR, Smith D, DeFronzo RA. The effect of growth hormone on glucose metabolism and insulin secretion in man. J. Clin. Endocrinol. Metab. 55:973–982, 1982.

53. Adamson U, Warren J, Cerasi E. Influence of growth hormone on splanchnic glucose production in man. Acta Endocrinol. 86:803–812, 1977.

54. Wilson DM, Baker B, Hintz RL, Rosenfeld RG. Subcutaneous versus intramuscular growth hormone therapy: Growth and acute somatomedin response. Pediatrics 76:361–364, 1985.

55. Kastrup KW, Christiansen JS, Andersen JK, Orskov H. Increased

growth rate following transfer to daily subcutaneous administration from three weekly intramuscular injections of human growth hormone in growth hormone deficient children. Acta Endocrinol. 104:148–152, 1983.

56. Prudden JF, Nishimara G, Ocampo L. Studies on growth hormone III. The effect on wound tensile strength of marked postoperative anabolism induced with growth hormone. Surg. Gyn. Obs. 107:481–482, 1958.

57. Barbul A, Rettura G, Prior E, Levenson SM, Seifter E. Supplemental arginine, wound healing and thymus: Arginine-pituitary interaction. Surg. Forum 29;93, 1978.

58. Wilmore DW. The metabolic management of the critically ill. Plenum, New York, 1977.

Index

Fat mobilization, role of GH in, 76
Free fatty acids
  effect of GH on, 75–104
  identity, 76

GHRH, 115, 119, 124–127
Glucocorticoids
  in GH lipolysis, 77, 81
  treatment with, 136
Glycerol, 76–104
  production increase, 89
G proteins, 79
GRF, 220–221
Growth
  catch-up, 141
  definition, 65
Growth hormone
  "bioinactive," 154, 159
  concentration, mean 24-hour in
      Turner syndrome, 198
  deficiency, 132–133
    "classical," 151, 156, 165
    diagnosis of, 145–191
    transient, 156, 159
    in Turner syndrome, 198
  diabetogenic activity of, 64,
      67–68
  direct actions, 28–31
    on adipose tissue, 29–30
    on carbohydrate metabolism,
        31
    on liver, 30
  excess
    effects of, 169
    height in, 183
  feedback mechanism, 35

growth-promoting activity of,
    63–70
indirect actions, 25–54
  on cartilage, 33
  on muscle, 31–33
insulinlike activity of, 64, 67–
    68
lipolytic effects of, 77, 81
neurosecretory dysfunction,
    151, 156
radioreceptor assay, 166
receptors, 1–17
reserve, 122–127
secretion
  in aging process, 222–224,
      227, 231, 238–239
  androgen, response to, 156–
      157
  arginine tolerance test, 159
  in genetic short stature, 180
  GHRH and, 127
  in humans, 119–122
  insulin tolerance test, 159
  neuroendocrine regulation of,
      113–127
  physiological properties of,
      258
  in rats, 115–119
  sleep and, 163
  stress, effects on, 258–260
  throughout day, 146
  12-hour nocturnal, 153, 158
  24-hour, 153, 158
therapy, 145–191
  administration of, 265
  bone maturation, 136, 139
  in catabolic states, 255–267
  ethical questions, 188–191
  growth rates on treatment,
      135

About the Editor

Louis E. Underwood is Professor of Pediatrics at the University of North Carolina School of Medicine, Chapel Hill, with which he has been affiliated since 1967. The author or coauthor of some 190 articles, reviews, book chapters, and abstracts, he has coedited or coauthored four books, and made lectures or presentations at conferences throughout the world. His research interests include the hormonal control of growth, growth hormone action, and the somatomedins. Among the professional organizations of which he is a member are The American Pediatric Society, The Endocrine Society, Lawson Wilkins Pediatric Endocrine Society, and Society for Pediatric Research. Dr. Underwood received the A.B. degree (1958) from the University of Kentucky and the M.D. degree (1961) from Vanderbilt University.